Linda's

Flat Stomach Secrets

Linda Lazarides

Other works by Linda Lazarides

Principles of Nutritional Therapy
The Nutritional Health Bible
The Waterfall Diet
Treat Yourself with Nutritional Therapy
The Amino Acid Report
The Big Healthy Soup Diet
A Textbook of Modern Naturopathy

About the Author

Linda Lazarides is a naturopathic nutritionist and founder of the British Association for Nutritional Therapy and Applied Nutrition. She has worked as a naturopathic practitioner for the British National Health Service and is best known for her work on water retention, described in her book *The Waterfall Diet* (Piatkus Books, UK bestseller).

©Linda Lazarides 2010
www.health-diets.net

Linda Lazarides asserts the moral right to be identified as the author of this work.

This publication may not be transmitted, in any form or by any means, electronic, mechanical, photocopying, recording or otherwise, without the prior permission of the publisher.

Disclaimer
This book is not intended as a substitute for proper medical advice. All persistent symptoms should be reported to a doctor.

CONTENTS

Introduction: Can you see your toes?
How I was inspired to create a recipe and begin the search for flat stomach secrets ....Page 4

Chapter 1
The way you walk can make you fat. Learn the walk that can make you tall and flatten your silhouette. Plus, the tummy exercises that work, and those that don't ....Page 8

Chapter 2
Learn about the 'alien within' and the common food ingredient which inflates your waistline by disrupting your hormones and giving you food addictions. Why you should not turn to 'diet' products to help you lose weight ....Page 16

Chapter 3
When your tummy is swollen and bloated. Learn about the effects of histamine, intestinal plaque, the side effects of gluten, and the bacteria that can make you look fat ....Page 39

Chapter 4
Water retention can masquerade as fat. Are you chubby, or just puffy? There's a difference. Beware of very low calorie diets: a lack of protein can give you a very swollen tummy ....Page 49

Chapter 5
Linda's Flat Stomach Diet. Put it all into practice with a simple meal plan and get the gorgeous silhouette you deserve .Page 63

Chapter 6
Linda's Internal Cleansing Routine. Here's what I did to help me see my toes again ....Page 73

Appendix I Recipes ....Page 76

Appendix II Vitamins A and D..Page 95

Appendix III Testing for problem foods.........................Page 98

Appendix IV Resources..Page 100

Can You See Your Toes?

In this book you will find out some startling and astonishing facts that few people know. Some of the secrets you will learn include:
- The difference between 'belly bulge' and 'belly flab'.
- You have a natural internal corset of muscles which you can strengthen while you're walking, driving or sitting at a desk.
- There is one common food ingredient which adds to your bulge more rapidly than anything else.
- Obsessive food cravings can come from a nasty type of fat that grows deep inside your tummy.
- Women who are most susceptible to stress have the biggest waistlines.
- Why consuming 'diet' products may make you *gain* weight.
- What causes bloating and gas and how to get rid of them.
- How eating a very low-calorie diet can give you a swollen tummy.

Everybody wants a flat tummy. Most of us look longingly at pictures of men with six-packs and models in bikinis with wonderfully toned midriffs. We sigh and shake our heads at the amount of work it takes to achieve such physical perfection. If only we had the time, energy, willpower and so on.

If you're anything like me, you might get motivated from time to time. Going on a diet, running, cycling or swimming or a subscription at the gym. Maybe the pounds start dropping off the rest of your body. But months later, when your willpower is mostly exhausted, more often than not your tummy is still nearly as large as ever, your toes are still invisible unless you pull your tummy in, and powerful control garments seem like the only remaining option. If only it was just a matter of losing a few pounds and doing a few sit-ups!

An episode from my past

In fact, getting a flat stomach could be easier than you think. I was inspired to write this book after recalling an episode in my life when my stomach became flat and I could see my toes with no problem at all. This happened when I was 20 years old, on a student trip in Romania. There were about 200 of us from many different countries, living in a large hall of residence, and all eating the same meals. It was a hot summer, and the inevitable struck—mass gastroenteritis. After two days of running to the lavatory six times a day, I suddenly noticed that my stomach was flat. Completely and wonderfully flat as never before!

Sadly, as soon as I recovered, my tummy went back to its normal bulging self. For the next 30 years I wondered how I could get my tummy flat again. I tried every kind of 'colon cleanse' routine, and even resorted to colonic irrigation—having my colon washed out with water twice a week for six weeks. Some people believe this approach works like magic. Not in my case! Nothing really seemed to help.

Finally, two years ago, after some self-experimentation, I created my Internal Cleansing Routine. After following it for three months, I could finally see my toes. The details of this routine are being published for the very first time in this book.

Easy, three-pronged approach

This guide would not be complete if all I did was give you my internal cleansing routine. It worked for me, but it's not the only solution. So I extended my quest to discover *all* the reasons why a tummy bulge can be so hard to lose. On my journey I found some extraordinary, sometimes horrifying, information which I'm sharing with you in this book.

After putting all this information together, I have designed a three-pronged approach to tackle the four main causes of tummy bulge. I believe it will massively improve your prospects of getting a lean and beautiful silhouette. My Flat Stomach Programme is designed for individuals who:

- Don't want to spend hours in the gym every week
- Have already spent hours exercising and still have a problem
- Don't want to starve themselves to lose weight
- Have a problem with bloating.

The three-pronged formula consists of:

- Exercises you can do while you sit or walk
- My Flat Stomach Diet
- My three-month Internal Cleansing Routine

Go ahead and get a beautiful body. Let me know how you get on!

Linda Lazarides

Success is a journey,
not a destination.
Focus on the process.

Chapter 1

The way you walk can make you fat

Nothing reveals your personality and hang-ups more than your posture and the way you move your body: the way you sit, stand and walk. Most of us don't walk very well. We waddle, slouch, march or strut. Dominant people stride purposefully, lead with the chin, or even seem to stamp as they walk. Less confident people drag their feet or shuffle along.

Many of us walk around leaning forward and partly

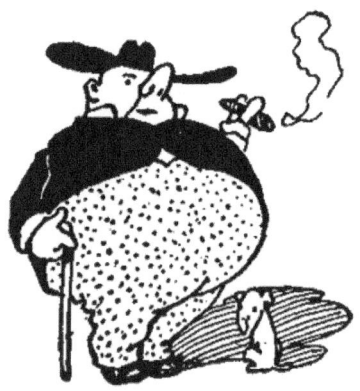

collapsed at the waist. Not only does this give you terrible posture, it makes your tummy look much larger than it really is, it makes you look older and it sets you up for back problems in later life. Try observing people as they walk. See if you can recognise your own gait or way of walking. By habitually using the wrong muscles when they walk, many people develop unshapely legs, or foot or back pain in later life.

Chapter 1

The Supermodel Walk

Few people, with the exception of those who've studied the Pilates exercise system or the Alexander technique for posture, have actually been taught the correct way to walk. But one profession—the modelling profession—has learned to make walking an art form. There's more to the model's walk than just looking elegant. It may surprise you to know that the catwalk style of walking uses exactly the right posture to help you get a flat stomach. Most aspiring models are probably not even aware of this, and may be spending time in the gym toning their tummies, not realising that they could be getting good results just by doing a lot of walking.

Of course it's not just supermodels who are trained in runway walking, but I'm going to call it the Supermodel Walk since that sounds cool and is easy to remember. The most important feature of the Supermodel Walk is to lift yourself up at the waist. Think about increasing the distance between your hips and the base of your ribs. Keep your ribs lifted as high as you can away from your hips, and your shoulders down and relaxed. Don't force your shoulders back or tense any other part of your body, but do lift up your neck and stand tall. Imagine you have a book balanced on top of your head. Practise this new posture for a few minutes, breathing in and out. It may feel a bit strange at first.

Now practice the walk

Keeping yourself lifted up at the waist, raise one foot straight in front of you as if starting to walk, but don't put your heel down yet. First put down the front of your foot (toes and ball of foot together) and then the heel. As your foot goes down and you lift the other leg to continue walking, you will feel some muscles deep down in your tummy working very hard to support you in this new posture. This may be a new sensation for you. The muscles you can feel are your transverse abdominals. They are deep 'core' muscles which, when toned, act like a corset for your tummy. Most of us don't use these muscles enough.

Next check your breathing. You should find that you are breathing out as your tummy muscles engage and breathing in as you lift your foot. (You don't need to breathe in and out with every step - normally there will be several steps to each breath.) As you take in breath, make sure that your tummy relaxes and feel your ribs expand under your armpits.

If you don't feel your deep abdominal muscles getting a workout, you are probably leaning forward too much. Try leaning back a little as you walk. Don't worry if it feels odd—it won't look odd at all. You will just look straight and upright. You have probably got used to leaning forwards as you walk. Leaning forwards makes you use your back muscles instead of your tummy. This will put an unhealthy strain on your back and give you a flabby front. Leaning forwards is tempting when you are walking uphill, but try not to do this. Stay upright and take smaller steps if necessary to reduce the strain. As your core muscles develop strength, the strain will get less.

That's all there is to the basic Supermodel Walk. Of course you will need to practise. It's a new sensation and it takes a bit of time to get it right. You'll soon find that not only does the Supermodel Walk give you better balance, it also gives your core muscles a work-out every time you walk. These muscles

Chapter 1

are exactly the ones you need to tone up in order to get a flat stomach. By lengthening your waist you also produce the immediate illusion of having a flatter stomach.

THE ABDOMINAL MUSCLES

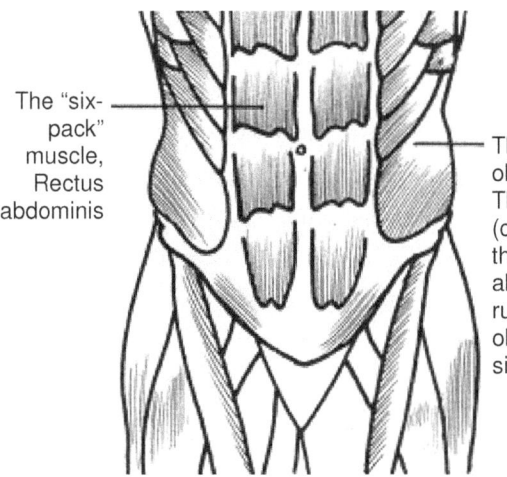

The "six-pack" muscle, Rectus abdominis

The abdominal oblique muscle. The deepest (core) muscle is the transverse abdominal which runs under the oblique and the six-pack.

The good thing about walking is that we can all manage to do a bit more without having to make a special effort. So that eliminates the problem of the gym subscription, swimming pool membership or exercise bike that never gets used. Just find a way to reduce motorised transport and replace it with 20 minutes more walking every day, and you will get results with very little effort.

'Core' is for corset

Now that you have discovered your core muscles, use them whenever you can. Engage them whenever you stoop down, lean or reach out. Use them to anchor your body whenever you change your centre of gravity. They are called the core muscles because they lie deep down, underneath your 'six-pack' muscle. The core muscles stretch all around your abdomen, acting like a corset to hold in the contents of your tummy (see how large an area they cover in the diagram on page 11). Just as your shape is instantly improved by wearing an elastic corset, the same will happen when you develop the strength of your core muscles to do the same job. Much of what you think is belly fat is really the bulge which you get when your internal organs are not properly supported by your core muscles. These muscles really are the key to a flat stomach.

The Belly-Button Scoop

I have adapted the Supermodel Walk to include a powerful tummy-toning exercise known as the Belly-Button Scoop or Ab Vacuum. This is done as you breathe out. Practise the Supermodel Walk for a while and get confident with it. Then, as you breathe out while walking, draw your belly-button towards your spine with a strong upward scooping motion, while still keeping your waist as long as possible. It's one of the best exercises for both the six-pack muscle and the core muscles. In fact you can do it all day long if you want—whenever you remember. This exercise can be done while sitting at a desk, in a car or while walking. Hold the scoop for a count of five to get even better results.

Chapter 1

You don't need a six-pack to get a flat stomach

When you go to the gym you probably learn to do sit-ups and crunches to exercise your abs. Many of the exercises you learn at the gym help to develop a 'six-pack'. A well-developed six-pack muscle (known as the Rectus abdominis) looks great, especially on men, but it is not enough to flatten a tummy bulge. It is the most superficial of your tummy muscles, and is used when you bend your body forwards. Most Rectus abdominis exercises don't work the deeper core muscles underneath.

The Pilates exercise system

If you're interested in learning more, consider taking up Pilates exercise classes. Pilates is different from body-building and general fitness regimes. It is mainly used for body shaping and sculpting, and is popular with many performing artists—actors, dancers and singers as well as models—to develop the strength, posture and body shape they need for their work. The Pilates system concentrates first and foremost on developing 'core strength'. In fact Pilates instructors always look so good that their body shape is referred to as the 'Pilates Body'. Yoga is also an excellent way to build core strength

In Appendix IV you will find links to YouTube videos with some short, simple Pilates routines for you to try.

More about your abdominal muscles

A study carried out at San Diego State University recently compared 13 common abdominal exercises in order to find which ones really do strengthen the abs. Many exercises (and devices used to help with exercising) were found not to be very effective. The bicycle crunch exercise came in at the top of the list of best exercises for the six pack and also works out the obliques.

How to do the bicycle crunch exercise

- Lie flat on the floor with your knees bent, feet on the floor, hands behind your head
- Stretch your left leg out and as you do so, bring your right knee and left elbow together
- Repeat with your left knee and your right elbow
- Repeat this cycling movement ten times, breathing evenly throughout the exercise.

www.ehow.com/video_2351933_bicycle-crunch-exercises-abs.html
The internal and external oblique muscles are located on either side of the Rectus abdominis. They allow sideways bending and twisting, and compression of the abdomen. A good exercise for the obliques is the reverse crunch.

How to do the reverse crunch

- Lie on your back with knees bent, feet on the floor and hands under your tailbone
- Breathe in, bringing your knees up towards your chest, lifting your bottom about an inch off the ground as you do so
- Keeping your knees bent, breathe out, contracting your abs as you do so, and lower your legs, but without touching the floor. Be careful not to use your back

muscles to take the strain. Your abs must do all the work.
- Repeat 2 and 3 ten times.

www.ehow.com/video_2351676_reverse-ab-crunch-exercises.html

The transverse abdominals are deep muscles located under the obliques and under the six pack. They cover a large area from front to back and from the ribs to the pelvis. Their fibers run horizontally, like a corset. These muscles are used when you expel air from your lungs. They stabilize your spine and help compress your internal organs. The already-mentioned 'belly-button scoop' primarily targets the transverse abdominals.

The psoas muscle, which runs from front to back in your hip area is very important to help stabilize the joint between your spine and pelvis. Damage to this joint (known as the sacro-iliac joint) is a major cause of lower back problems.

Visit **www.health-diets.net/flat-stomach/members/** for clickable versions of all the internet links in this book.

Chapter 2
Beware the alien within!

We all know about the fat on the outside of your stomach, that you can pinch between finger and thumb. Have you ever wondered why the size of your waist doesn't seem to match the amount of fat you can pinch? I used to know a woman named Maggie who was overweight probably by about 30 lbs. One day I saw her in a bikini and was completely amazed that her stomach was absolutely flat, even though it had a bit of fat on it.

Only recently have I discovered how that is possible. There are actually two kinds of tummy fat. One is external (the fat you can see and hold on to). The other is internal. Internal fat is also known as 'visceral fat'. It accumulates inside the abdomen, between the internal organs, and makes the belly protrude or stick out at the front. Maggie's stomach was flat because she had very little internal fat.

A tummy with a lot of internal fat is also known as a 'pot-belly' or sometimes a 'beer belly'. If you have this problem, you can measure how severe it is by calculating your 'waist to hip ratio'. The higher the ratio, the more internal fat you have.

Calculate your waist-to-hip ratio (WHR)

You will need a measuring tape and a calculator.
1. Gently breathe out and relax.
2. Without holding in your tummy, measure your waist circumference. (Your waist is at the halfway point between the base of your ribs and your hip-bone.) You can use inches or centimeters. Do not pull the tape too tight.

This chart assesses your health risks based on your WHR

Men	0.95 or less	low risk
	0.96 to 1.0	medium risk
	1.0 or higher	high risk
Women	0.80 or less	low risk
	0.81 to 0.85	medium risk
	0.85 or higher	high risk

3. Measure your hip circumference around the fullest part of your bottom.
4. Using your calculator, divide the waist measurement by the hip measurement.

For example, if your waist is 36 inches and your hips are 42 inches, then divide 36 by 42. The answer is 0.85, which is your waist-to-hip ratio.

People with a high WHR are considered to be at risk of getting a heart attack, stroke or diabetes. The WHR is thought to predict a person's risk of these problems more accurately than their overall body weight or even their body mass index (BMI). Not only that but fat accelerates ageing, probably by speeding up the unravelling of basic genetic structures inside cells. Writing in the medical journal the *Lancet* in 2005, Professor Tim Spector and his colleagues at St Thomas' Hospital, London, and at the University of Medicine and Dentistry of New Jersey, studied more than 1,000 women, and found that the more people weigh, the older their cells look. Obesity adds the equivalent of almost nine years of age to a person's body, and smoking has similar harmful effects.

Why is internal fat like an 'alien being'

It's bad enough that internal fat expands your waistline. But this type of fat also has some nasty 'alien' characteristics.

- Like an alien being, internal fat protects its own growth and development at your expense by giving you addictive food cravings. It does this by deactivating a substance called leptin which your body produces when you've had enough to eat. (NB: fructose, a sugar which we will discuss later, can also deactivate leptin.) Without sufficient leptin you feel hungry all the time.
- Internal fat also protects itself from destruction by disrupting your hormones. When it reaches a certain critical mass it forces your body to step up production of the hormone known as insulin. Insulin protects this fat and prevents it from being broken down and used for fuel.

The more internal fat you have, the closer you are to developing high blood pressure and diabetes. Nothing predicts these diseases better than your waist size. If your waist circumference is more than 40 inches (100 cm) then you so close to developing these problems that you may already have them.

More harmful effects

The 'alien' analogy is not so far off. Scientists really *are* saying that internal fat can take on a life of its own. Unlike the fat under your skin, internal abdominal fat is highly active, a living, throbbing organ that produces particles which attack good health. These particles are known as cytokines. They cause inflammation and swelling and are blamed for a wide range of health problems from heart disease to diabetes, dementia

Chapter 2

(senility) and rheumatoid arthritis. In fact, internal fat is so strongly linked with diabetes, that in animal experiments carried out at the Albert Einstein College of Medicine, New York, in 2002, the pre-diabetic condition known as 'metabolic syndrome' was reversed when the animals' internal fat was cut out and removed.

What Causes Internal Fat?

Stress

So far we know of two main causes. The first is a hormone produced by your adrenal glands (situated above your kidneys). Its name is cortisol and it helps your body to cope with stress.

Researchers have known for some time that people with Cushing's syndrome—a disease in which levels of cortisol are very high—seem to have very large waistlines due to large amounts of internal fat. In healthy people, cortisol levels rise when they are under stress. Although all of us are exposed to stress, some people produce more cortisol than others. Also, some people become stressed more easily than others, or fail to learn to adapt to stressful situations. In 2000, Dr Elissa Epel and her colleagues at Yale University decided to investigate whether people who get stressed very easily, have larger waistlines.

Dr Epel measured the WHR of 59 women and, over a period of several days, gave them laboratory stress tests and then tested the amounts of cortisol they produced when they were under stress. About half the women had a high WHR and the other half had a low WHR. The results were astounding. Women with the biggest waistlines did indeed seem to get stressed more easily and produced more cortisol than women with a smaller waistline.

The researchers concluded that women who are more nervous, or more vulnerable to stress, are more likely to find that their waistline expands as they get older. This happens even if they don't consume any more calories, and even if the rest of their body is not particularly fat.

Of course, genetics, other hormones and lifestyle can also play a role. Smoking, alcohol and lack of exercise tend to increase internal fat, say the researchers, whereas getting sufficient sleep and exercise can help to reduce it. Their findings were reported in the journal *Psychosomatic Medicine* in 2000.

Sleep also helps to slow down the ageing process. People who don't sleep enough have higher levels of the cytokine proteins which we now know to be key promoters of diabetes and heart disease.

Other hormones

Internal fat starts to affect men in middle age when their testosterone levels go down and their oestrogen (estrogen) levels go up. Men with a lot of internal fat are often said to have a 'beer gut'. Alcohol does indeed play a big part in the development of internal fat since it decreases the ability of the liver to break down oestrogen. When oestrogen is not broken down it circulates in the body and can encourage both internal fat and the development of 'man boobs'.

Men with a zinc deficiency may also be prone to developing these problems, as a lack of zinc encourages testosterone to turn into oestrogen. Overall body weight plays a part too. Testosterone in overweight men gets converted to oestrogen more rapidly.

In women, on the other hand, oestrogen seems to offer some protection against the development of internal fat, as this type of

Chapter 2

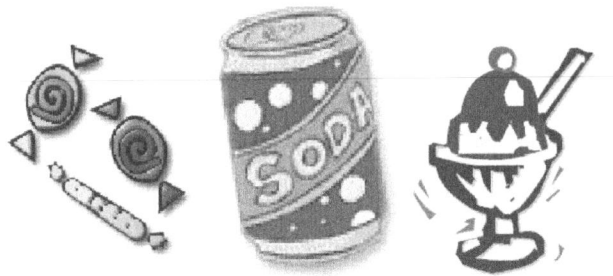

fat mostly develops after the menopause, when oestrogen levels decline and the proportion of male hormones rises. Before the menopause, women store fat in their hips and thighs, but after the menopause, fat migrates to their belly.

Sugar and insulin

Many of us turn to sugary foods when we are under stress, even though we all know that sugar is a very concentrated source of calories and liable to make us put on weight. Any sugar which your body cannot use gets turned into fat quite quickly.

Most of the sugar we consume is hidden in sugary foods and soft drinks or sodas. It's very easy to put on a lot of extra weight if you indulge in these foods and don't take enough exercise to burn off the extra calories.

When you consume sugar, it's not just the calories that make you put on weight. A much more serious fattening effect comes from the hormonal and metabolic changes that take place. Consuming sugary foods and drinks makes you produce insulin, and the more sugary the items you consume, the more insulin you produce. Consuming foods which are high in both fat and sugar, such as chocolate and ice cream, makes you produce even more insulin.

Insulin makes you put on weight because it increases the amount of fat that goes into storage and stops you breaking down fat to use as energy.

Types of sugar

As we know, fat can go into storage under your skin, or inside your abdomen, (internal fat). The amount of internal fat you store depends on the type of sugar you consume, so it's time to learn a few things about sugar.

The sugar crystals that you buy in packets or which are added to food usually consist of a chemical known as sucrose. Sucrose itself consists of two individual sugars bound together, whose names are fructose and glucose. When you eat sucrose, you are eating 50 per cent glucose and 50 per cent fructose—half and half. Your digestion breaks the sucrose down into these two individual sugars which then enter your bloodstream.

Glucose travels around your body and can be used as fuel or turned into fat. But fructose does not travel around. It stays in your abdomen, and your liver turns it into internal abdominal fat.

This discovery is quite recent. In 2009 doctors Stanhope and Havel at the University of California carried out research in which they asked two groups of people to drink beverages every day in addition to their normal diet. The first group had to drink beverages sweetened with glucose and the other group had to drink beverages sweetened with fructose. After ten weeks, both groups had gained the same amount of weight. But while the glucose group gained fat evenly throughout their body, the fructose group were found to have gained substantially more internal fat.

Chapter 2

Does sugar really give you energy?

Many people believe the old saying that sugar 'gives you energy'. But US bodybuilding and fitness guru John Parrillo has discovered that fructose actually robs you of energy. It does this by forcing your body to turn some foods into fat instead of turning them into glycogen, the carb you need to fuel your muscles. When muscles lack glycogen, you feel heavy and lethargic. When your muscles have plenty of glycogen, you feel energetic and full of stamina.

Parrillo's experiments

Parrillo has carried out many nutritional experiments with bodybuilders. When a bodybuilder gets close to a contest, his (or her) body fat levels get so low that any tiny change becomes immediately apparent and is easy to measure. This state is ideal for experiments, so Parrillo has been able to measure the effects of many different foods. In one of his early tests he removed 300 calories-worth of rice from the bodybuilders' daily diet and replaced it with 300 calories-worth of bananas—a sugar-rich fruit. To his amazement the athletes started to gain fat. He continued the experiment for two weeks and they continued to gain fat. Then he stopped the bananas and put the rice back in. The fat started to reduce.

These results were mind-blowing, as they thoroughly explode the myth that calories are calories and the type of calorie makes no difference to your body weight.

Complex carbs are best

Parrillo knew that in order to work, muscles need glycogen, which is a form of carbohydrate that they can store and utilise as

> In the mid 1980s manufacturers started mass sweetening of soft drinks with high-fructose corn syrup (HFCS). It's very cheap, very sweet, and it's 55 to 90 per cent fructose.
> **'The increased use of HFCS in the United States mirrors the rapid increase in obesity.'**
> *American Journal of Clinical Nutrition, April 2004*

fuel. If you want to feel energetic and burn off the calories in your food rather than turn them into fat, you have to eat carbs that drip-feed glycogen into your muscles. Complex carbohydrates such as bread and rice (preferably whole-grain), pasta, potatoes, beans and oats are very good at this, as they are broken down and absorbed slowly.

On the other hand if you consume a soda or drink sweetened with corn syrup, or eat something sugary, the fructose in these items will hog the enzyme which turns carbs into glycogen. Fructose uses the enzyme to turn itself into glycogen for the liver, but that glycogen can't be used by the muscles. (The liver can't use very much of it either.) So for the next few hours the muscles will get less glycogen, even if you have just done a workout and your muscles are weak and starved. The unused liver glycogen becomes internal fat, and the carbs that could not be made into muscle glycogen are also made into fat. Result? More fat, less energy.

How To Reduce Internal Fat

Controlling Fructose

It you want to lose tummy fat and gain energy, it's clearly very important to avoid eating fructose-rich foods as much as possible. This means you have to check the labels of everything

Chapter 2

you consume. Most sweetened products such as ice cream, chocolate and desserts will have 'sugar' listed in their ingredients. Sugar usually means sucrose, which as we know is half glucose and half fructose. It's not good, but there are sweeteners out there with even higher amounts of fructose. In recent years there has been a tendency to use corn syrup as a sweetener. It's very cheap, has a lot of sweetening power, and consists of 55 to 90 per cent fructose. Sometimes known as HFCS (high-fructose corn syrup) it is found in a wide variety of commercial, processed foods, especially soft drinks or sodas.

Fructose is often claimed to be a healthy option because it has a low glycaemic index—it doesn't raise blood sugar very much. But the reason for its low glycaemic index is that your liver quickly turns it into fat.

Another so-called healthy option, agave nectar, is actually 56 to 92 per cent fructose, depending on the brand. Even honey is mostly fructose.

Recommended fruits

All fruits contain fructose (another name for fructose is fruit sugar) but the following fruits are recommended more than

Sweeteners and their glucose and fructose contents

Food	Fructose (grams/100 g)	Glucose (grams/100 g)
Sucrose	50	50
Honey	40.9	35.7
Corn syrup	55 to 90	10 to 45
Agave nectar	56 to 92	8 to 44
Maple syrup	50	50

others, as they have the least amount of fructose:
- Stone fruits: apricots, nectarines, peaches, plums
- Berry fruits: blueberries, blackberries, boysenberries, cranberries, raspberries, strawberries
- Citrus fruits: kumquats, grapefruit, lemons, limes, mandarins, oranges
- Other fruits: ripe bananas, jackfruit, kiwi fruit, passion fruit, pineapples, rhubarb, tamarillos.

Apples and pears are fine to eat, as they contain only a few grams of fructose. But you may wish to avoid their juices, which are quite high in fructose (some canned fruit products are canned in pear juice).

Artificial sweeteners

If you intend to improve your waistline but are not ready to take up meditation or knitting instead of comfort food to relieve stress, you will have to find an alternative sweetener.

Artificial sweeteners may appear to be the answer, and perhaps they are ok if consumed in small amounts, very occasionally. Personally I would never eat or recommend these chemical products. I believe they cause stress to the liver, and can be difficult to metabolise. Some, such as aspartame—the chemical name for proprietary sweeteners used in hundreds of 'low-calorie', 'sugar-free' or 'diet' products—have been linked with unpleasant health problems such as dizziness, recurring headaches and even seizures.

There's also new research to show that artificial sweeteners can intensify cravings for sweets and other carbohydrates. Incredibly, researchers have found that food and drink containing these sweeteners can lead to faster weight gain than sugary foods and drinks.

A 2008 Purdue University study published in the journal *Behavioral Neuroscience*, reported that rats fed with artificially-sweetened yoghurt gained more weight than rats given yoghurt containing natural sugar. The rats which were fed artificial sweeteners ended up eating more and adding extra body fat compared with the rats whose yoghurt was sweetened with glucose sugar.

Humans gain more weight too

But it's not just animals who suffer these effects. A major American research study was carried out in 1988 on 80,000 women aged 50 to 69 years. Those who used artificial sweeteners were compared with those who did not. Regardless of their initial weight, the women who used the sweeteners put on more weight per year than the women who did not use them. (Reported in *Appetite* journal, Vol 11, 1988.)

Increased appetite

It seems that sweeteners may make you put on weight because they increase your appetite. Another study was carried out in 1990 at the Monell Chemical Senses Center, Philadelphia. For 15 minutes, 10 men and 10 women chewed gum sweetened with four different doses of aspartame. Their subsequent hunger was then compared with groups given either nothing or unsweetened gum. The gum containing the least aspartame did not significantly increase appetite, but the gum containing moderate amounts did. The gum containing the largest amount of aspartame initially reduced appetite but this was followed by a sustained increase in hunger cravings. (Reported in *Physiology and Behavior* journal, volume 47, 1990.)

Hunger cravings are due to insulin

Researchers have been trying to explain why this hunger occurs. It seems that your gut has 'taste' cells which taste sugar and artificial sweeteners through the same mechanisms used by the taste cells on your tongue. The gut's taste cells regulate the secretion of insulin and hormones that govern appetite. Whether you eat sugar, or whether you just eat something that tastes like sugar, your body produces similar amounts of insulin. The insulin searches for the expected sugar, but when it is not found it eliminates some of your blood sugar instead. As your blood sugar drops, you develop hunger cravings which then make you eat more. (*Artificial Sweeteners: Fat or Fiction*? International Institute for Anti-Ageing http://bit.ly/XSEg.)

The ideal sweetener?

When searching for the ideal sweetener, I looked once again to the world of bodybuilding and the experiments of John Parrillo. Parrillo has been hailed as an exercise and nutrition genius who knows more about losing body fat and maximizing muscle energy than anyone else in the world. I knew that if his recommendations met the stringent requirements of world-class athletes then they would work for anyone. John's advice is simple. Use a sweetener which breaks down only to glucose, not to glucose and fructose.

Glucose itself is no good as a sweetener because it rushes too quickly into the bloodstream and pushes up insulin levels. The muscles can't use all that glucose straight away, so the remainder gets turned into fat. A much better sugar to use as a sweetener is maltose, which is the sugar found in a carb known as maltodextrin, and also in rice or barley malt syrup. Maltose consists of two molecules of glucose, but the glucose has to be extracted by digestive enzymes, so is released gradually. You can buy snack bars sweetened with rice dextrin or maltodextrin (look for them in the sports section of your local health food store) and you can buy brown rice syrup or barley malt syrup to sweeten other foods or drinks.

Brown rice syrup—a slow-release carb

Brown rice syrup is made by culturing rice with enzymes to break down the starches, then straining off the liquid and cooking it to a syrup. The final product is roughly 50% soluble complex carbohydrates, 45% maltose, and 3% glucose.

Maltose takes up to one and a half hours to be digested, and the complex carbohydrates take from two to three hours, so brown rice syrup is a good slow-release carb for replenishing muscle glycogen.

John Parrillo has one more piece of advice. To avoid turning your maltose into fat, consume it after a workout or other physical exertion when your muscle glycogen stores are depleted and need to restock themselves. If you make these suggested changes, you could find that your muscle health, instead of continuing to decline as you get older, improves and gives you the energy to exercise more and burn off more fat.

Exercise

The next most important step to reducing internal fat is to get more exercise. Exercise gets rid of internal fat more quickly than any other fat, and the older you are, the more quickly it goes. Scientists believe that exercise achieves this positive effect by breaking down fructose more rapidly, and by increasing levels of growth hormone. Growth hormone suffers at the expense of the high cortisol and high insulin levels that come with a large waistline. People with a deficiency of growth hormone tend to have less flesh and more body fat, especially internal body fat.

How to increase growth hormone with exercise

In one study, male participants were put through endurance training 5 days per week for 6 months. When compared with the young participants, the elderly ones showed a 20 per cent greater reduction in internal fat even though they started off with twice as much internal fat as the young men. To raise your growth hormone levels you need to spend at least 10 minutes exercising at a level that gets you out of breath. Multiple daily 10-minute sessions help to keep your growth hormone levels high during the day. Getting sufficient sleep helps to keep up growth hormone levels at night.

Special advice for men

As we already know, testosterone seems to be protective against the development of internal fat. But too much alcohol, combined with a zinc deficiency, can reduce testosterone and increase oestrogen levels in men. To prevent the decline of testosterone, first and foremost you need to cut right down on alcohol and ensure that your diet has plenty of zinc-rich foods: whole-grains, fish and seafood. Other important foods to consume every day are the Cruciferous family of vegetables: broccoli, cauliflower, cabbage or brussels sprouts. These will help you break down and excrete oestrogen before it can act on your body's tissues. Next in importance come parsley, celery and thyme—good sources of a flavonoid known as apigenin. Apigenin partly blocks the aromatase enzyme which converts testosterone into oestrogen. You would need to consume a lot of apigenin to make a substantial difference, but adding these foods to your diet is a step in the right direction. Hesperidin found in orange peel, also helps to inhibit the same enzyme.

To help you relax and sleep, drink chamomile tea or take Passiflora herbal tablets before you go to bed. Both are good sources of chrysin—another substance which helps to block the aromatase enzyme.

Special advice for women

Women are much more prone to developing internal fat after the menopause, when oestrogen levels decline and levels of male hormones rise. Some foods are rich in gentle plant oestrogens, which can help to rebalance a woman's hormones and help her lose weight from around her waist. In 2007 scientists at the University of Alabama gave a group of 15 menopausal women a daily soy-rich drink for three months. Another group of similar women received a dummy treatment. At the end of the three months, the soy-treated women had lost fat around their waistline, but the group on the dummy treatment had gained fat. (This research study was reported in the journal *Fertility and Sterility*.) In this study the scientists measured the fat under the women's skin (their subcutaneous fat) rather than their internal abdominal fat, but soy is probably also capable of reducing internal fat. The beneficial substance found in soy is known as genistein, and it works by acting on insulin. As we know, people with a lot of internal fat tend to produce more insulin. This insulin protects fat from being broken down and used as fuel, but genistein from soy can block the protective effect.

Some years ago the media threw doubt on the value of soy as a health food. If you would like to consume more soy products but are worried about these doubts, please read the special note on soy at the end of this chapter.

Oestrogen after the menopause

It is not widely known that women produce male hormones in their adrenal glands, which are situated above the kidneys. Normally these male hormones are made into oestrogen by means of an enzyme called aromatase. This process continues after the menopause, and ensures that women continue to have a source of oestrogen. The aromatase enzyme can be damaged by smoking and by vitamin or mineral deficiencies, so it's important to look after this important enzyme and give it what it needs to do its job.

So far, scientists have identified two nutritional deficiencies which can hinder the work of aromatase: vitamin D and boron. Vitamin D is produced in your body when your skin is exposed to sunshine. Few foods contain vitamin D, other than liver and full-fat dairy products such as butter and cheese. In these modern times when we stay out of the sun and eat low-fat foods, we are at risk of vitamin D deficiency. There is no supplement which I recommend more frequently than cod liver oil. This is mostly because it is a good source of vitamin D, but also because it is one of the few sources of ready-made vitamin A— another nutrient which is at risk of deficiency if you eat a low-fat diet. See Appendix II for more about these two vitamins.

Boron is a mineral found mostly in vegetables. Studies have shown that women who don't get enough boron in their diet may have lower oestrogen levels. Boron also helps to protect the bones of menopausal women, by preventing them from excreting too much calcium.

Licorice

The natural herbal product licorice actually encourages the aromatase enzyme to produce oestrogen from male hormones. But licorice also has other benefits if you are trying to lose internal fat. Scientists have become very interested in researching this herb, which is used as a flavouring in the West but as a medicine in the Far East. They have found that a flavonoid substance called glabridin in licorice can help to control the amount of internal fat produced in your body, and also boosts the activity of enzymes which break down internal fat. In a randomized, double-blind, placebo-controlled trial, overweight people were supplemented with 900 mg per day of licorice extract for 12 weeks. There was a substantial decrease in internal fat as well as an overall decrease in body weight.

The researchers used very powerful licorice extracts. You have to be careful with anything this strong, especially as consuming too much natural licorice can raise your blood pressure. But women can certainly drink licorice tea and take licorice supplements which have had the potentially harmful component removed. See Appendix IV for where to get these products.

Another useful herb, especially for menopausal women, is Agnus castus, sometimes known as 'chasteberry'. Agnus castus helps to maintain a healthy balance between the two main female hormones, oestrogen and progesterone.

Oestrogen and breast cancer

After the menopause, many cases of breast cancer, as well as fibroids, are caused by high levels of oestradiol, the most potent form of oestrogen. The liver breaks oestradiol down to less potent forms and so protects a woman from its cancer-promoting effects. But in order to provide this protective effect, she needs to eat foods which help her liver to make the enzymes it needs. Every woman should consume vegetables from the Cruciferous family several times a week. These vegetables include broccoli, brussels sprouts, cabbage and cauliflower.

Drink Tea To Lose Weight

Both black and green teas contain a substance known as epigallo-catechin gallate (EGCG) which helps to increase your sensitivity to insulin. When you are properly sensitive to insulin, your body does not make such large amounts of this hormone, so there is less risk of getting metabolic syndrome—the prediabetic condition caused by high insulin. As we know, too much insulin also protects internal fat from being broken down, so keeping down insulin levels is doubly desirable. The beneficial effect of tea is lost if you add milk, so you should drink your tea green or black. *Journal of Agricultural and Food Chemistry, 2002, 50 (24), pp 7182–7186. Research carried out at the U.S. Department of Agriculture.*

The Grapefruit Diet Is Not A Myth

Scientists at the Pennington Biomedical Research Center in Louisiana fed a group of overweight people half a fresh grapefruit before each meal to see if they would lose weight. After 12 weeks, they lost 1.6 kg, compared with the group on the dummy treatment, which only lost 0.3 kg. The grapefruit also seemed to improve insulin sensitivity in those members of the group who suffered from metabolic syndrome.

Chapter 2

A special note about soy

Soy is clearly a good food to help women lose body fat. But it has taken quite a battering in the press over its safety for animals and young children. The question-marks mainly hang over its potential to raise oestrogen levels, the possibility of harmful effects on the thyroid gland, and possible effects on mineral absorption and protein digestion.

Oestrogenic effects

Substances known as 'isoflavones' in soy products, can mimic the effects of oestrogen. In one study, pregnant Rhesus monkeys who were fed concentrated soy isoflavones developed abnormally high oestrogen levels. But research on human women who are given natural soy foods instead of these concentrated extracts, does not show these abnormalities.

Research into breast cancer prevention also shows mixed results, with some studies showing a protective effect from soy products, and others showing unhealthy changes to cells. Again, some of these studies were carried out using soy protein isolate (SPI) – a highly processed concentrate with very high levels of isoflavones. SPI is nowadays a very common ingredient in modern processed and fast foods, bakery products and diet beverages, and is used to make the 'meat substitute' known as textured vegetable protein (TVP).

Anti-thyroid effects in children

There are numerous reports of babies developing goitre after feeding with soy-based infant formula. Children raised on soy-based infant formula are twice as likely to develop a condition known as autoimmune thyroiditis, where the immune system attacks and destroys the cells of the thyroid gland. Some researchers believe that feeding babies with soy formula gives them the oestrogen equivalent of five contraceptive pills a day.

Phytic acid

Phytic acid in soy foods combines with minerals in our diet, and hinders their absorption. Phytic acid is also found in raw grains such as muesli, and in unleavened wholegrain bread such as chappatis. It can cause deficiencies of minerals such as iron and zinc. These effects can be prevented by combining soy with protein foods such as egg, meat and fish—which is the usual practice in oriental diets. But vegetarians who eat no animal products may be vulnerable to mineral deficiencies from phytic acid, so are advised to supplement with multiminerals if they consume soy products regularly.

Protease inhibitors

These are substances which inhibit protein digestion, and are found in soy and in raw pulses (legumes), grains, nuts and seeds. If we cannot digest our protein we cannot absorb vital amino acids. Protease inhibitors are normally broken down by cooking or by sprouting seeds. For instance, there are large amounts of protease inhibitors in raw muesli, which disappear if you soak the muesli in water for at least a few hours.

How much soy is it safe to eat?

Research is still scanty, so there's no real answer. It is probably sensible for adults to avoid eating highly concentrated soy products every day, and for young children to avoid them completely. TVP and SPI are also found as ingredients in many processed and fast foods.

Similarly, be cautious about taking supplements of genistein and daidzein—two of the most potent isoflavones in soy. Some women who have taken these supplements to prevent hot flushes have developed thyroid abnormalities.

The forms of soy which are not concentrated, are soy milk, tofu (or bean curd), soy yoghurt, miso, soy sauce, tamari sauce and tempeh. All of these except soy milk and tofu contain low levels of phytic acid, because they are fermented products. Phytic acid is much reduced by fermentation.

Soy milk contains four times the amount of protease inhibitor found in tofu. But I have known women who cured themselves of endometriosis by drinking half a litre of soy milk every day. Like fibroids and most breast cancers, endometriosis is caused by an oestrogen overload in the body. The weak plant oestrogens in soy attach themselves to oestrogen receptors in the body, helping to balance more potent human oestrogens such as oestradiol. The result is a healthier balance of oestrogen levels.

For women, it does not take a lot of soy to balance oestrogen levels. Half a litre of soy milk is about 2 cups or 16 fluid ounces, but this probably does need to be consumed at least 5-6 times a week.

A sensible soy intake for a woman?

On balance, as a woman, I would not hesitate to consume up to 2 litres of soy milk or soy yoghurt a week plus 2-3 portions of tofu and a little soy sauce. As a nutritionist I am convinced by the science that this would actually bring me health benefits and is not enough to cause any problems as far as my thyroid gland or the phytic acid or protease inhibitor content are concerned. My only concern is that many soy crops nowadays are genetically engineered. Like most consumers, I am very much opposed to this so I would certainly go for organic brands.

As we know, men are also prone to excessive oestrogen

levels, so natural soy foods may be beneficial for them too, but probably in smaller amounts than for women.

Alternative baby milk formula

On the other hand I do feel that soy is risky for babies and should also be limited for young children. If you have a baby who cannot be breast fed and is allergic to cow's milk formula, it's well worth considering a goat milk infant formula instead. These are available from

United Kingdom: http://amzn.ws/nannygoatformula-uk

United States: www.genesisorganics.com

Visit **www.health-diets.net/flat-stomach/members/** for clickable versions of all the internet links in this book.

Chapter 3

When your tummy is swollen and bloated

So far we've looked at how to use your muscles to keep your tummy flat, and how to cut down on internal fat. But another big cause of an expanded waistline—bloating—has nothing to do with fat or muscles. We all get bloated from time to time if we over-eat or get constipated or eat the wrong foods. But imagine what it's like to walk around bloated all the time? This is the reality for countless people—it's a huge problem.

Food-related bloating means that your intestines are irritated. It's as simple as that. Bloating in your abdomen is just the same process as getting a swollen finger from an insect sting, or a swollen nose from hay fever. The sting or the pollen causes an irritation, and your body tries to get rid of it by creating histamine which causes a swelling known as inflammation. Your finger eventually heals, but for your intestines that's more difficult, as the cause of the irritation can continue indefinitely.

The effects of histamine

Histamine widens the gaps between cells in your small blood vessels and your intestinal lining, so that extra fluid can get into the tissues. It's this fluid which makes the tissues swell up when they are inflamed. (Tissues just means the 'fabric' of your body, for instance muscle tissue, lung tissue, intestinal tissue.) The fluid brings white blood cells to the tissues, and these white cells try to gobble up whatever is causing the irritation. If they don't succeed, the swelling will continue.

Inflammation is meant to be an emergency measure. If it goes on for a long time in the intestines it can be quite damaging. Swollen intestinal membranes have difficulty producing enzymes and absorbing your food, so vitamin and mineral deficiencies can develop even if you eat a very good diet. When gaps widen between the cells of your intestinal lining it becomes leaky, allowing small particles of partly undigested food to enter your bloodstream and travel around your body. These particles should never be in your blood. They are very irritating, and so can force your body to produce histamine just about anywhere. This produces allergic symptoms like headaches, skin rashes and swollen, painful joints, and can also affect your kidneys.

In this chapter we will look at what can irritate your intestines so that we can stop the swelling and bloating, and help your tummy resume its normal shape.

What irritates the intestines?

There are three main causes of irritated intestines.
- Poor digestion
- Intestinal plaque
- Toxin-producing bacteria.

Digestion

We tend to take good digestion for granted, and only worry if we get heartburn or other severe discomfort. In fact lots of things can affect how well we digest our food, including stress, overeating, eating in a hurry, not chewing enough, drinking too much liquid with a meal, or taking antacid indigestion medicines. As we get older, the ability to make acid in our stomach tends to decrease. This can be a problem, as the presence of acid is needed to trigger off the rest of the digestive process. The stomach also needs acid in order to kill any harmful bacteria or parasites which we accidentally ingest with our food.

Some of us eat far too many of the foods which are hardest to digest, particularly gluten-rich foods, cheese and eggs. Even cows' milk protein is relatively hard to digest. When food is not properly digested, two things happen. First, mild irritation occurs in the lower part of the intestine. This part of the intestine is more sensitive to undigested food because—apart from dietary fibre—it is not supposed to come into contact with it. Secondly, the undigested food is seized and fermented by the hungry bacteria which normally live in the lower part of the intestine. When these bacteria get lots of food, they thrive, multiply and produce gas. If you get intestinal gas all the time even when you haven't been eating beans, it is very likely that your digestion is weak and a lot of fermentation is going on in your tummy.

Irritable bowel syndrome is a name given by doctors to a collection of tummy symptoms, including gas, bloating, griping pains, constipation and/or diarrhoea. It is often relieved by avoiding the hard-to-digest foods mentioned above. If you suffer from bloating, you might want to give that a try. If this approach is only partially successful, then poor digestion is not the only cause of irritation in your intestines.

Intestinal plaque

We have all heard of dental plaque—the sticky bacteria-laden deposit which rots your teeth and damages your gums. Naturopathic practitioners believe that it is possible to develop intestinal plaque too. Intestinal plaque (sometimes known as 'mucoid plaque') is also sticky and full of bacteria. Many naturopaths believe that it develops in the large intestine (colon) and can be removed by colonic irrigation—washing out your colon with water. Although some people can lose a lot of sticky material when they undergo a course of colonics, I am not at all sure that for most people the colon is the main location of this plaque. Anatomically-speaking, a far more logical place for it is the lowest part of the small intestine, because food deposits are more easily trapped there.

My view is that, like dental plaque, intestinal plaque consists of partly-digested food particles and millions of bacteria, and that it collects in between the little 'villi' whose job is to absorb your food. The stickiness is due to gluten-rich food particles. Just as in the mouth, the bacteria trapped in this plaque are likely to be 'anaerobic' bacteria which, because they live without oxygen, produce a lot of acid. This irritating acid is liable to damage the absorption surface of our small intestine, just as the acid from dental plaque bacteria damages our teeth and gums. The diagram on the next page shows the kind of progressive damage that takes place. The damage happens slowly, over many years, and as it progresses, bloating gets worse and it gets

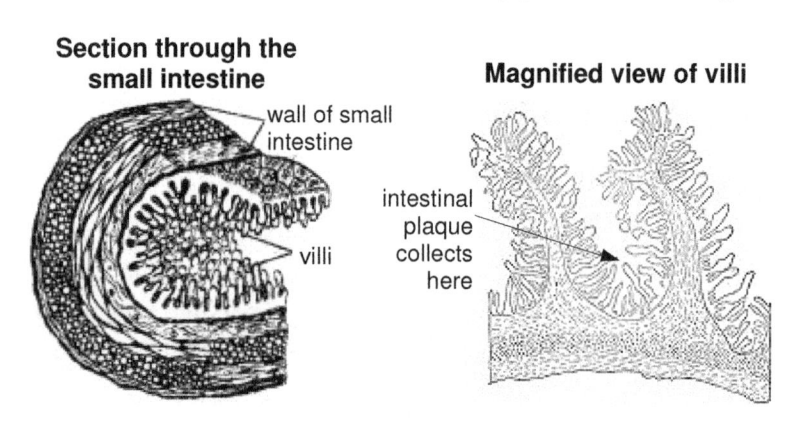

Section through the small intestine

wall of small intestine

villi

Magnified view of villi

intestinal plaque collects here

Chapter 3

Healthy villi: tight gaps between cells and plenty of absorption surface

bloodstream ———

Inflamed villi: wider gaps between cells and reduced absorption surface

bloodstream ———

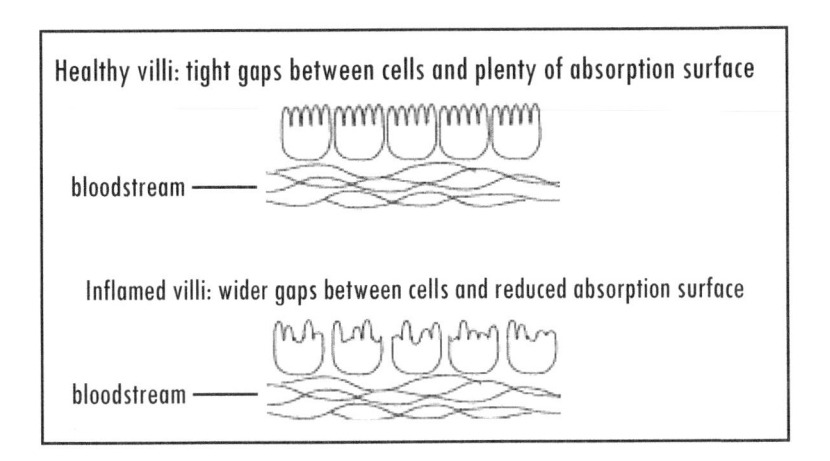

harder for you to absorb your food.

You are more likely to suffer from intestinal plaque if you habitually suffer from constipation, and eat a diet which is low in fibre and high in white flour products: white bread, cakes, biscuits, doughnuts and pasta. How many people do you know who eat toast for breakfast, sandwiches for lunch and pasta for dinner, with cakes and cookies or biscuits in between?

Gluten encourages intestinal plaque

Flour, and especially white flour, contains large amounts of gluten, a substance so sticky that when you mix flour with water you can stick wallpaper to your wall. Gluten is hard to digest and moves slowly through the digestive system. It is prone to collect between your villi and is hard to dislodge. In her book *A Matter of Life* (Macdonald Optima, 1990) medical doctor and biochemist Dr Nadya Coates advises everyone to cut down on gluten. Research units, tagging gluten with radioactive material, have shown particles of gluten escaping into the blood circulation through an irritated, leaky intestinal lining, and becoming embedded in joints, liver, spleen, pancreas or

Some gluten-rich foods

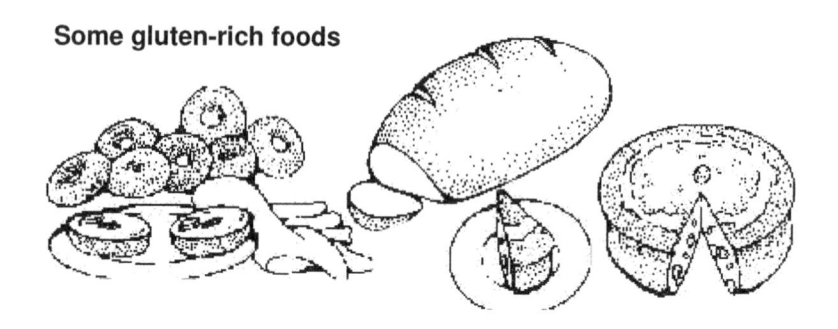

gallbladder. Over the years they are likely to cause arthritis or slow down the circulation and block the transport of nutrients and oxygen, especially in the brain.

A connection with Ayurvedic medicine

It is very interesting that Ayurvedic medicine—the ancient medicine system of India, which dates back thousands of years—blames many health problems on intestinal plaque, which it calls 'ama'. Even thousands of years ago Indian doctors knew that ama could leak out of the intestines and settle in joints, inflaming them and causing arthritis. A large part of Ayurvedic medicine is about getting rid of ama, which is said to be a result of 'reduced digestive fire'. Ayurvedic practitioners recommend reducing gluten-rich foods and consuming an anti-ama diet of foods which are easy to digest. Bitter foods are included to stimulate the digestive juices, and garlic, ginger and spices are recommended to control the growth of bacteria. Fasting is sometimes used as a treatment to 'digest' ama.

Gluten can make you feel sleepy

Gluten is also known to contain peptides (protein fragments) with an 'opium-like' effect. In one research study where wheat

Chapter 3

gluten was broken down into peptides and tested, some of the peptides produced morphine-like effects. Many people feel drowsy after a meal containing gluten, and children with autism often improve if gluten and milk are removed from their diet. If you sometimes feel drowsy after meals, it could be due to gluten. I now only eat gluten-rich foods occasionally, and have noticed that whenever I do, I need an extra 1-2 hours of sleep at night. When I've been gluten free for a few days, I feel much more alert and need less sleep.

In Chapter 6 you will find my Flat Stomach Diet to cleanse your intestines. But in the meantime it would be a good idea to think about some alternatives to toast, cakes and sandwiches.

Toxin-producing bacteria

Intestinal plaque is bad enough, but extremes of irritation and bloating can occur if our small intestine become colonised and overgrown with toxin-producing bacteria such as Clostridium, Klebsiella and Giardia, or yeasts such as Candida. Normally the so-called 'friendly' bacteria in our intestines help to control these microbes, but friendly bacteria are quickly destroyed by antibiotics. This leaves the field clear for antibiotic-resistant undesirables to take over, which they do with remarkable speed. Bacteria can divide and multiply every 20 to 30 minutes, which means that if 1,000 are present in your small intestine at 6 pm, by the time you get up at 8 am the following morning this figure may have risen to 16 million, and to countless millions by the morning after that. Over the years, large areas of your intestine can be colonised by yeasts and bacteria.

Probiotics

Many people who suffer from bloating are encouraged by TV advertising to eat 'probiotics'—yoghurt containing friendly bacteria. There is no harm in trying this if you want, but if you have a long-standing problem with bloating you have probably found that you don't respond quite as well to this treatment as you would like. These are really food products intended for an occasional bout of bloating. If you have a severe or long-standing case of toxic bacterial overgrowth, eating probiotics is a bit like throwing grass seed over a thick patch of weeds. To get rid of this problem properly takes several months of intensive anti-microbial therapy, followed by treatment with friendly bacteria products which have been developed for clinical use.

On the other hand it is very beneficial to eat probiotics every day if you are currently taking antibiotics. This will help to replace the friendly bacteria which are destroyed by these drugs, and prevent the antibiotic-resistant undesirables from getting out of control. Since antibiotics will deactivate probiotics if taken at the same time, wait an hour or two after taking antibiotics before you eat your probiotic yoghurt.

A new study reveals that the artificial sweetener Splenda (sucralose) reduces the amount of good bacteria in the intestines by 50%. Splenda alters gut microflora and increases intestinal p-glycoprotein and cytochrome p-450 in male rats. *J Toxicol Environ Health A*. 2008;71(21):1415-29.

Dysbiosis—the cause of many health problems

If your intestine is already overgrown with toxin-producing bacteria or yeasts, you have probably developed a number of health problems besides bloating and bowel problems, and have

Chapter 3

been searching for answers for a long time. This condition, which is known as 'dysbiosis' produces so many symptoms that doctors get very confused. The most common of these symptoms is feeling tired and 'hung-over' all the time, but the toxins from dysbiosis can also affect your glands, or give you asthma, arthritis or nervous problems. Most doctors are not trained to look for dysbiosis as a cause of these problems, so you may end up getting tranquillisers for your nerves, an inhaler for your asthma, antidepressants for your fatigue, and IBS medicines for your bloating. Unfortunately none of these treatments will really get to the root of the problem, which is a mild form of poisoning from toxin-producing bacteria in your intestines.

Healing your intestines

If you have not yet consulted a doctor, you are advised to do so. This book cannot take the place of proper medical advice. But if you have consulted a doctor and have been given the all-clear to try natural self-help methods, you will find helpful information in Chapters 5 and 6.

First of all, your diet need to be based on foods that are easy to digest and will not encourage congestion, irritation or the growth of undesirable bacteria. To help cleanse and sweep your small intestine, your stools need to be kept as soft as possible for about three months, with gentle laxatives and a suitable fibre supplement to bulk them up. Foods such as pineapple juice, ginger and garlic help to loosen sticky mucus which may be bound up with gluten deposits, and tea made from spices such as cinnamon, cloves and cardamom helps to control the growth of bacteria.

If you think you may have a problem with toxin-producing bacteria in your intestines, you can also try adding some food supplements which make your tummy a more hostile environment for bacteria and yeasts. These include bromelain (pineapple extract) and herbal extracts of oregano, cloves and wormwood. Bromelain supplements are taken with meals and the herbal extracts can be taken with the evening meal or as part of the Internal Cleansing Routine in Chapter 6.

Some people also find fish oil supplements helpful to control swellings and inflammation.

See Appendix IV for where to get the recommended items.

Chapter 4
Water retention can masquerade as fat

Your tummy can also be swollen by water. If you think you may have water retention, you first need to get the all-clear from your doctor before you start looking at natural treatments. Problems with the heart, liver or kidneys can cause water retention (usually in the form of swollen legs and ankles) which needs medical treatment. If your organs are pronounced healthy, then if you do have water retention, it can usually be helped by the kind of dietary changes recommended in Chapter 5.

Water retention is not just a major cause of tummy swelling (especially in women). By masquerading as fat it can also cause overweight. Many people with this hidden water retention try to lose weight by eating very little and exercising for hours every week. Unfortunately they often fail to get good results because a low-calorie diet has no effect on water retention. Very low-calorie diets can even make water retention worse by reducing your protein intake too much.

How can you tell if you have water retention?

It is sometimes hard to tell if your problem is water retention rather than just fat, but one of the main signs is that your weight will probably fluctuate a lot from day to day. Some people with water retention have to get up several times in the night to pee and then weigh several pounds less in the morning than they did the night before. Others find that one day they weigh 195 lbs and the next day 200 lbs. It is not possible to gain five lbs of fat in a single day, so this weight difference is probably water.

Another sign of water retention is when you are puffy rather

Symptoms of Water Retention

- ❏ Have you worked hard to lose weight using conventional methods, and found that you cannot get below a certain weight even if you persevere for months or years?
- ❏ Press a fingernail firmly into your thumb-pad. Does it stay deeply dented for more than a second or two?
- ❏ Press the tip of your finger into the inside of your shin-bone. Can your finger make a dent?
- ❏ Water retention often collects in the legs and ankles. Do your ankles ever swell up?
- ❏ Does your shoe size seem to increase as you get older?
- ❏ Do your rings sometimes seem not to fit you any more?
- ❏ Do you get a major swelling problem in hot weather?
- ❏ Water retention can cause bloating. Is your tummy often tight and swollen?
- ❏ If you are a woman, do you often suffer from breast tenderness?
- ❏ If you are a woman, do you gain weight pre-menstrually?
- ❏ Does your weight ever fluctuate by several pounds within the space of only 24 hours?

If you can answer Yes to two or more of these questions, there is a strong possibility that you may have a water retention issue.

Chapter 4

than flabby. Fat tends to hang off you in folds, whereas water makes your skin look more rounded or puffy.

It may also be a sign of water retention if you regained a lot of lost weight very quickly after stopping a low-carb diet. Some of the foods which are not allowed on a low-carb diet are prone to causing water retention. When you stop eating them you can lose water weight very quickly. As you reach your target weight and jump for joy, it is only natural to put the diet aside and resume normal eating. But only too often all the lost water weight will return within a few days.

Swollen legs and ankles, swollen tummy, painful swollen breasts, difficulty getting rings on and off your fingers—any of these can be signs of water retention.

You might be able to control water retention temporarily by taking diuretics (herbs or medicines that make you pee more). But if you want to stop your water retention from coming back you need to find out what is causing it so that you can work on eliminating the cause.

Protein deficiency

A protein deficiency can give you a tight, swollen belly as shown in the picture of the little African boy on the next page.

To prevent water from collecting in your tummy you must eat enough protein. In fact, most people eat too much protein rather than too little—we only need a few ounces a day. Dieticians have recently announced that people in the Developing World can get enough protein for their daily needs just by eating a lot of rice. Of course that is not an ideal diet by any means. I am only intending to illustrate that you can still eat more protein than you need even if you have little money.

In the Western world, the people who are at risk of suffering from water retention due to protein deficiency are:
- Those on Very Low Calorie Diets (VLCD) of less than 1,000 Calories* a day,
- People with anorexia nervosa,
- Strict vegetarians (vegans) who are not eating enough protein-rich plant foods such as rice, nuts and beans.

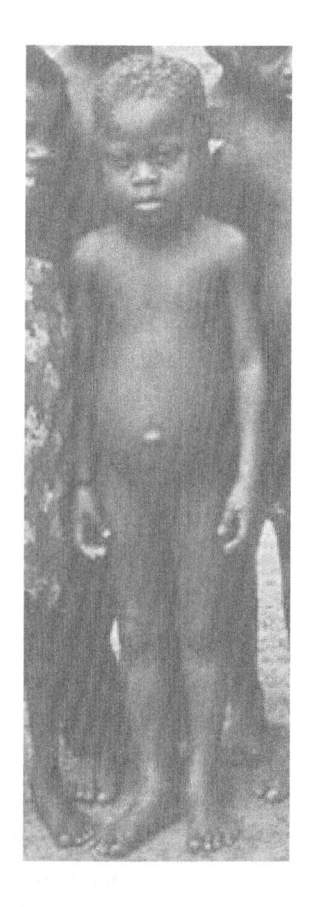

This little African boy is suffering from malnutrition. He is not getting enough to eat, and the lack of protein is causing severe water retention in his tummy, while his arms and legs remain very thin.

*1 Calorie is equivalent to 1,000 calories or 1 kcal

Chapter 4

VLCD (Very Low Calorie Diets)

If followed for months or years, VLCD of less than 1,000 Calories a day can lead to water retention just because the dieter is eating so little food that his or her protein needs are not being fulfilled. The ironic thing is that people who already have water retention may start a VLCD because they believe their weight problem is due to excess body fat. When they find that the VLCD does not produce the desired weight loss, they persevere with the VLCD on a long-term basis, and the lack of protein results in even worse water retention and consequent weight *gain*.

These are very sad cases and real psychological damage can occur. I have known people who became pathologically afraid of eating normal food portions because the link between calories and overweight has been so firmly fixed in their mind for so long. Yet if they do not stop the VLCD and eat more, they risk gaining even more water retention and developing other problems such as chronic fatigue, low sex drive or even an abnormal heart rhythm.

And don't forget that long-term VLCDs (as well as "yo-yo" dieting) can also make you gain weight more easily by slowing down your metabolism by up to 45 per cent.

Strict Vegetarians

Most vegetarians are very sensible about ensuring that they get enough protein. But any person who is grappling with a long-term weight problem can in time become less sensible. I have occasionally known vegans (strict vegetarians who consume no animal products, not even milk or yoghurt) who have tried to live for years on plain steamed vegetables and green salad without dressing.

This approach is a form of VLCD, but one extremely lacking in protein. If followed for months or years it may lead to the thin arms and legs and large belly that we all associate with Third World malnutrition. The matchstick arms and legs of malnutrition are caused by the body breaking down its own tissues to get some protein to feed its vital organs. The large belly is in fact swollen with water retention.

A dieter with this problem can become totally irrational and simply does not accept that the large belly size is due to eating too little rather than too much. We are not used to seeing this body pattern in the West, and we do not associate it with self-inflicted starvation. People with anorexia nervosa are very vulnerable to this problem.

Other nutritional deficiencies

Vitamin and mineral deficiencies in the Western world are much more common than we think. The problem is that most of us eat quite large amounts of foods which have had most of their vitamins and minerals removed, for example:

- White flour, white pasta, white bread etc.
- White rice
- Sugar (both brown and white), as found in candy, cookies, chocolate and confectionery, ice-cream, desserts and soft drinks.
- Refined vegetable oils
- Other fats as found in desserts, bakery and patisserie products, ice cream, potato chips and crisps, mayonnaise, dips, deep-fried foods etc.

If 50 per cent or more of the calories you eat come from these foods, then you are only getting 50 per cent of the vitamins and minerals that you could be getting from a more natural diet.

Chapter 4

How do you know that this is enough to make all the hormones, blood cells, electrolytes, nerve transmitters and so on that you need? The answer is that of course you don't know. Minor symptoms of nutritional deficiencies such as skin rashes and spots, fatigue, split or brittle fingernails, mood swings, irregular heartbeats and palpitations, premenstrual syndrome, nervous problems, memory problems and so on, are widespread. If we are deficient enough in vitamins and minerals to show these symptoms, then our water balance is almost certainly also at risk.

Take a look at some of the older members of your family who have the same dietary habits as you, who take the same amount of sugar in their tea and coffee, and so on. Do they have any health problems? When you look at them, you are looking at yourself a few years down the line. A lot of the health problems which have been attributed to inherited 'genetic' factors are actually due to inheriting dietary habits. If you can start to develop more healthy habits you may be able to prevent not just water retention, but other problems too.

Several nutrients are especially important to maintain a healthy water balance:
- B vitamins
- Magnesium
- Iron
- Vitamin C and flavonoids

B vitamins

Vitamin B6 is especially important to prevent water retention. This vitamin is mostly found in whole-grain bread, wheatgerm, pumpernickel bread, brown rice, oats, nuts, sunflower and sesame seeds, avocado pears and bananas. If you don't eat some of these foods every day, you could be at risk of deficiency. Alcohol consumption can aggravate a deficiency as it inactivates vitamin B6. The contraceptive pill and hormone-replacement therapy also inactivate vitamin B6.

I come across people with vitamin B6 deficiency all the time, and I am not alone. In a British research study carried out in 1981, 17 per cent of pre-school children were found to have B6 intakes below the recommended daily amount.

If you don't get enough B6, your body will suffer from these problems (among others):
- Reduced ability to absorb protein from your food
- Reduced absorption of magnesium into your cells
- Higher levels of hormones which slow down water excretion. In women this is often worse pre-menstrually, and causes tummy bloating and swelling.

Other B vitamins are important too. A lack of B vitamins widens the joins between cells in the walls of your small blood vessels. This makes them leaky, allowing water to collect in your tissues.

A woman's liver needs enough B vitamins (as well as Cruciferous vegetables such as broccoli and cabbage) to break down potent forms of oestrogen which can otherwise linger and cause water retention.

Magnesium

While playing just as important a role as calcium in the body, magnesium remains the poor relation who gets little attention from doctors and dieticians. Magnesium is mainly found in whole-grain bread, pumpernickel, brown rice, oats, nuts, sunflower and sesame seeds, soybeans and leafy green vegetables. If you neglect to eat a variety of these foods every day you are really playing Russian Roulette with your body's

Chapter 4

water balance.

Coffee is one of magnesium's greatest enemies; one of the reasons why drinking too much coffee can make you nervous and twitchy is that coffee makes you excrete magnesium in your urine. Other enemies of magnesium include consuming too much fat and protein (as in some low-carb diets) and living a high-stress lifestyle.

If you don't get enough magnesium, your body will suffer from the following problems which can lead to water retention:
- Lower potassium levels
- Sodium accumulation
- Higher levels of aldosterone, a hormone which slows down your kidneys.

The high blood pressure (known as pre-eclampsia) which can occur in pregnancy, is due to low magnesium levels causing water retention. Extra water in your tissues tends to raise your blood pressure, and the extra nutritional demands of pregnancy can aggravate a borderline magnesium deficiency.

Iron

Most people know that a lack of iron leads to anaemia (anemia). Anaemia causes oxygen starvation and an overworked heart. Oxygen can only be absorbed from your lungs if your red blood cells contain enough iron. With a lack of iron, your heart has to work extra hard trying to get your blood to your lungs as frequently as possible. When overworked for many years, a heart becomes less efficient, and this can lead to water retention. A lack of zinc, vitamins B6 or B12, folic acid or the amino acid taurine can also cause anaemia. Iron deficiency also makes your thyroid gland less efficient. Your thyroid governs your metabolism.

Vitamin C and flavonoids

Flavonoids are the dark red, blue and purple pigments found in fruits such as black cherries and blueberries. With the B vitamins and vitamin C, they help to maintain the proper structure of blood vessel walls, preventing them from leaking too much fluid into the tissues.

Foods that affect your kidneys

Salt, through the sodium it contains, plays a special role in how your body fluid behaves. When sodium rises in your blood, (due to eating salted foods), you get thirsty and drink more to dilute this sodium. Your kidneys will not release the extra fluid until you eat less salt. I have known heavy salt consumers who lost three lbs weight within a few days just by giving up salt. This extra weight was all water.

You can reduce your salt intake by avoiding salty and smoked foods, by being cautious with all foods not prepared at home (especially if they taste salty), and by using low-sodium salt or salt substitute in cooking and at the table.

Since your kidneys have to excrete water, their health is very important. If your kidneys are sick, urination is reduced and water retention increases, especially in the legs and ankles. Two things which are very damaging to the kidneys are a deficiency of the mineral selenium (found in sea fish and Brazil nuts) and an excess of a metal called mercury, found in amalgam (silver) tooth fillings.

Research from the University Hospital of South Manchester in England shows that high levels of insulin are also bad for the kidneys. Insulin is produced at higher levels when you consume sugary foods and drinks.

Histamine

As we know, if your intestinal lining is irritated or leaky, it can allow particles of undigested food to get into your blood. As these particles circulate they are treated as foreign invaders, making your body produce histamine. Histamine makes small blood vessels leaky, allowing extra water to enter your tissues. Some foods, especially gluten-rich foods, egg and dairy products, are more difficult to digest and so are more prone to causing this problem. If you have this problem and eat the wrong foods every day, your tissues may not get the chance to release this water, and may develop permanent water retention.

People whose small intestine is very irritated and leaky can have problems with numerous foods. Researchers at the Henri Mondor Hospital in Créteil, France, have found that these histamine reactions can affect the kidneys, which become inflamed and stop working properly, causing water weight to accumulate. Once the problem foods are identified and withdrawn from the patient's diet, the kidneys work normally again and the water is rapidly shed by urination over the next few weeks.

Removing the problem foods is helpful in the short term, but in the long term people with this problem really need a treatment to help heal their irritated intestines.

Diuretics (medicines which stimulate the kidneys to work harder) should never be used to treat water retention caused by histamine or nutritional deficiencies. By dehydrating the blood they could aggravate a water retention problem.

Toxins and medicines

Our bodies are exposed to toxic substances all the time, from airborne pollutants to pesticides and bacterial toxins absorbed from our intestines. When toxins are absorbed, some cells in our body may accumulate them more than others. For instance toxins found in plastics can lodge in blood vessel walls, causing inflammation and swelling.

There are many things we can do to help our liver break down toxins and our intestines eliminate them. The liver needs B vitamins, protein and antioxidants. Certain herbs and spices—for instance milk thistle and turmeric—can give it much-needed support. Vegetables in the Cruciferous family (broccoli, cabbage and brussels sprouts) help the liver to break down excessive amounts of oestrogen, which in women can encourage water retention, breast tenderness, fibroids and endometriosis.

Prescription drugs which can cause water retention include many blood pressure medications, pain-killers and anti-inflammatories. Some of the main categories include:

- Beta-blockers
- Calcium-channel blockers
- Clonidine
- Methyldopa
- Insulin
- Metoclopramide
- Oral contraceptives and HRT/ERT drugs
- Steroids
- Some NSAIDs (non-steroidal anti-inflammatory drugs)
- Danazol

More information can be found in my book the *Waterfall Diet*, published by Piatkus Books and available from bookstores and

Chapter 4

Amazon websites. You will probably know these medications by their brand names so if you are not sure what you are taking, try searching on the Internet to find out if your medication falls into one of these categories.

Exercise

Periods of inactivity, such as
- Bed rest (invalids or post-surgery cases)
- 'Couch potato' lifestyle
- Long-distance flights

can lead to water retention in your tissues. This is because the drainage network in your body (the lymphatic system) can get sluggish when you are not moving around. If you have a tendency to water retention, you should get as much exercise as you can.

Raw vs. cooked food

There is no doubt that raw food is very healthy and many people thrive on it, especially if they live in a hot climate. But very little raw food is eaten in the Far East, and traditional Chinese medicine actually teaches that too much raw food can encourage weight gain. It is all to do with the balance of Yin and Yang, the two opposing energies that drive our metabolism.

I have always found that eating salad to lose weight leaves me feeling even more hungry. In my experience, hot foods are much more sustaining. Best of all is soup, which is both filling and low in calories due to the high liquid content. If you haven't already discovered it, you might be interested in my book the *Big Healthy Soup Diet* published by Thorsons, and available from Amazon websites.

In the oriental system of medicine, the main cause of

overweight is held to be water retention, which cools down the metabolism and prevents fat loss. The Chinese recommend several foods to help get rid of water retention, including broad beans (and tea made by adding boiling water to dried broad bean pods) aduki beans and mung beans. They also recommend increasing Yang energy in the body by eating liver, kidneys, fish and seafood. Garlic, ginger, chives, and particularly cinnamon are also considered to be very helpful for losing weight.

Diet to help water retention

The Flat Stomach Diet in Chapter 5 is designed to combat most aspects of water retention as well as bloating.

Chapter 5
The Flat Stomach Diet

Now it is time to apply all the dietary recommendations from chapters 2-4. The basic principles of Linda's Flat Stomach Diet are simple: eat from List A frequently, avoid the foods in List B,

List A: Foods and drinks to consume frequently	
Aduki, mung and broad beans	In Chinese medicine, considered to help prevent weight gain by preventing water retention
Celery	Combats water retention. For men helps to slow down conversion of testosterone to oestrogen.
Cinnamon	Helps control intestinal bacteria. Chinese remedy to prevent water retention and weight gain
Cloves	Help control intestinal bacteria
Cruciferous vegetables: broccoli, cabbage, cauliflower	Help to break down potent forms of oestrogen. Good for men to help prevent internal fat, good for women to help prevent water retention
Garlic	Helps to loosen intestinal plaque
Ginger	Helps to loosen intestinal plaque
Grapefruit	Helps to improve sensitivity to insulin
Green tea	Helps to improve sensitivity to insulin
Licorice tea	Boosts activity of enzymes which break down internal fat
Oily fish (salmon, sardines, mackerel etc.)	The oils help to combat inflammation and premenstrual bloating. These fish are also a good source of zinc.
Parsley	Combats water retention. For men helps to slow down conversion of testosterone to oestrogen.
Pineapple juice	Aids digestion. Helps to loosen intestinal plaque.
Radish juice	Good for the thyroid. Helps loosen intestinal plaque.
Seafood (prawns, shrimps, shellfish)	Rich in zinc, which helps men keep up testosterone levels. Boosts Yang energy, to aid weight loss.
Soy foods (soy milk, soy yoghurt, tofu)	Help to allow the breaking down of internal fat by blocking the effects of insulin

List B (the 'no' List): Foods and drinks to avoid

Apple and pear juice	High in fructose
Alcoholic drinks: beer, wine, spirits	Alcohol increases internal fat. In men increases conversion of testosterone to oestrogen
Dairy products: milk, cheese, butter, cream, yoghurt*	Potential triggers of bloating or water retention
Dried fruit	High in fructose
Eggs and foods containing traces of egg*	Potential triggers of bloating or water retention
Foods and drinks sweetened with sugar or honey. All sweeteners except brown rice (malt) syrup.	High glycaemic index or high in fructose
Foods containing yeast: bread, fermented products, foods containing yeast extract*	Potential triggers of bloating or water retention
Gluten-containing foods: bread, cakes, biscuits, cookies, pasta, and any foods containing wheat, oats, barley or rye. Check all labels carefully.*	Potential triggers of bloating or water retention. May encourage intestinal plaque formation.
Saturated fats, including hydrogenated fat and red meat (beef, pork, lamb)	These fats harden the outer membranes of red blood cells
Salt and salty foods such as smoked fish. Also sodium-rich items such as baking powder	Excess salt and sodium cause water retention

*Avoid these foods completely for four weeks

and eat all other foods in moderation. Please take a look at the two lists now, read the notes, and then check out the suggested Seven-Day Meal Plan.

Note on potential triggers of water retention

These foods do not in themselves cause water retention, but individuals who do not digest them well may find that they trigger this problem. If you lose a lot of water weight during the recommended four weeks of avoidance, you are probably one of these individuals.

To find out which of these foods you can safely resume

Chapter 5

eating, you need to carry out the self-test in Appendix III. This test involves reintroducing the starred foods one by one, while monitoring your weight and how you feel. NB: You cannot carry out this test until you have cleared all residues of the starred foods completely out of your system, by totally avoiding them for four weeks. Read all labels carefully!

Note on saturated fat

Not only do the forms of saturated fat listed opposite tend to raise cholesterol levels, they congest your liver and harden your cell membranes, making it harder for red blood cells to squeeze through narrow blood vessels, bringing oxygen to delicate tissues such as brain, eyes and ears. Also, since large amounts of internal fat are stressful for your liver, it makes sense, while you are trying to lose this fat, to avoid eating forms of fat which raise your cholesterol, slow down your circulation and cause additional stress to your liver.

Seven-Day Meal Plan

A Seven-Day Meal Plan is provided on pages 66 to 67, but you do not have to follow it. You can simply eat from List A, avoid the foods in List B, and eat all other foods in moderation. The Seven-Day Meal Plan is meant to be very basic and very simple to give you ideas for preparing quick, simple meals. It helps you to get the balance right, and hopefully will give you techniques and ideas for putting together your own quick, healthy meals.

You will notice that evening meals in the meal plan are mostly based on soup. This is to help you lose weight. As explained in my book the *Big Healthy Soup Diet* (Thorsons, 2005) research shows that eating soup reduces the appetite for subsequent meals. Because of the liquid content, soup also

The Seven-Day Meal Plan

Day	Breakfast	Lunch
Monday	Pineapple juice, green tea, gluten free cereal with soy milk and chopped almonds	Piece of cold chicken with salad of roasted peppers, tomatoes and courgettes (zucchini) with olive oil, balsamic vinegar and orange or lemon zest. Cinnamon tea.
Tuesday	Grapefruit, green tea, gluten free cereal with soy milk and chopped Brazil nuts	Chickpea salad with parsley, chopped celery, chopped red onion and French dressing. With rice or corn cake(s) and a scraping of pure olive oil spread. Cinnamon tea.
Wednesday	Beet(root) juice, green tea, gluten free cereal with soy milk and sunflower seeds	Canned sardines with salad of cooked brown rice tossed with French dressing, chopped parsley, celery, red and green peppers. Cinnamon tea.
Thursday	Grapefruit, green tea, gluten free cereal with soy milk and chopped walnuts or pecans	Aduki bean salad with parsley, chopped celery, tomato and French dressing. With rice or corn cake(s) and a scraping of pure olive oil spread. Cinnamon tea.
Friday	Pineapple juice, green tea, gluten free cereal with soy milk and chopped cashew nuts	Prawns (shrimps) in egg-free mayonnaise with salad of cooked brown rice tossed with chopped parsley, celery, grated radish and French dressing. Cinnamon tea.
Saturday	Green tea Smoothie: soy milk, avocado, ground almonds (almond flour) and fresh or frozen berries Kedgeree with peas and haddock	
Sunday	Green tea Smoothie: soy milk, avocado, ground almonds (almond flour) and fresh or frozen berries Fish fillet fried in olive oil with grilled (broiled) courgettes (zucchini) and tomatoes.	

See Appendix I for the recipes

Chapter 5

Dinner

Celery and radish juice
Yellow lentil, potato and cauliflower soup with coriander (cilantro) spiced with curry powder
Soy yoghurt with fresh or cooked fruit
Ginger or cinnamon tea

Celery and radish juice
Broad bean, broccoli and chicken soup
Soy yoghurt with fresh or cooked fruit
Ginger or cinnamon tea

Celery and radish juice
Green lentil soup with white fish, cabbage, ginger and chives
Soy yoghurt with fresh or cooked fruit
Ginger or cinnamon tea

Celery and radish juice
Red lentil soup with broccoli and chicken
Soy yoghurt with fresh or cooked fruit
Ginger or cinnamon tea

Celery and radish juice
Mung bean soup with onion, garlic and tofu chunks
Soy yoghurt with fresh or cooked fruit
Ginger or cinnamon tea

Celery and radish juice
Thai chicken curry with chopped vegetables, coconut milk and rice noodles
Rice pudding with fresh or cooked fruit
Ginger or cinnamon tea

Celery and radish juice
Gluten-free pasta bake with salmon and roasted vegetables
Tofu chocolate mousse
Ginger or cinnamon tea

satisfies the appetite with fewer calories.

If you lack ideas of your own, you can repeat the Seven-Day Meal Plan as often as you wish—back-to-back until you reach your target weight. It is not necessary to stop it after seven days.

Possible side-effects of the diet

Most people will start to feel clearer and lighter after a few days on this diet. But before this you may experience some temporary tiredness, headaches or lethargy—usually due to cutting out coffee, alcohol or other foods which you have been consuming frequently.

Intestinal gas may be a problem if you are not used to eating a lot of beans, lentils and vegetables. Consuming double-strength spice teas (cinnamon and cloves) with meals can help to relieve this.

Occasionally some individuals are sensitive to soy products. If the diet is still making you feel unwell after a week you may be one of these. Try cutting out soy to see if that makes a difference. Soy milk can be replaced with rice or nut milk.

Snacks

Proper meals are recommended, since when you eat snacks it is easy to pile on the calories without realising it. Suitable snacks include
- Leftover soup
- Any of the breakfast or lunch items in the Seven-Day Meal Plan
- Almonds or sunflower seeds
- Peanut butter or hummus with rice cakes, corn cakes (similar to rice cakes) or raw vegetable sticks

Chapter 5

- Soy yoghurt with fruit
- Rice pudding made with soy milk and sweetened with brown rice syrup or malt syrup.

Drinks

As explained earlier, green tea, licorice tea (for women only) and spice teas can actually have value as weight loss aids, so I recommend that you drink these in preference to other beverages. Ginger tea is one of the best possible digestive aids. Teas are best unsweetened, but brown rice (malt) syrup can be used occasionally as a sweetener.

If you need to relax (for instance before bed-time) have a cup of chamomile tea. This is especially good for men as it helps to inhibit the enzyme that turns testosterone into oestrogen.

You should also drink two litres (eight glasses) of water a day. Water absorbs the most waste matter from your blood and helps to carry it out of your body. Other drinks do not have such cleansing power. For instance, imagine washing your face in coffee or cola!

With the exception of apple and pear juices, fruit juice is also a suitable drink, but should be diluted half and half with water in order to reduce the fructose content. To make a delicious natural fruit soda drink, use sparkling water as a mixer. Grapefruit juice and pineapple juice do not need to be diluted, as you are consuming them for therapeutic reasons.

Vegetable juices can have enormous medicinal value. The benefits of celery and radish juice are described on page 63. Beet(root) juice is rich in iron and can help to boost energy levels.

Frequently asked questions

Q. How soon will the Flat Stomach Diet work?

This varies depending on your age, state of metabolism, how much water weight you are carrying, and how much work you need to build up the strength of your natural 'corset' (core muscles). The younger you are and the worse your previous dietary habits, the faster the diet will work. If you are over 45 years old, don't be discouraged if results seem slow at first. Your body just needs time to repair its metabolism.

Q. How strictly do I need to follow the diet?

I recommend following it very strictly for four weeks. Even small lapses can undo some of the benefits on your hormones and water balance in the early stages.

Q. I am a vegetarian. Is there a meat-free version of the diet?

If you do not eat fish or chicken, you can substitute a handful of nuts or a portion of tofu in these recipes. Nuts can be ground in a food processor or with a hand-held rotary grater. When added to a bean or lentil dish such as soup, the amino acids from nuts combine with the amino acids from beans or lentils to make a complete protein.

Q. Can I swap the meals around?

There is no problem with changing the order of the meals.

Q. I don't like some of the foods. Can I leave them out?

You can leave out anything you want, but in that case you may have to reduce your expectations of what the diet can do for you. If you think of foods as medicines it may be easier to cope.

Q. What sort of quantities should I eat?

In general, you should eat just enough to feel satisfied. Eat slowly and chew well so that you don't accidentally get past this point without realising it. If you have a history of overeating,

Chapter 5

pay special attention to portion control. Calorie-counting is beyond the scope of this book, but in general women trying to lose weight should eat no more than 1,500 kcal per day and men no more than 2,000. Observe the plates of slim people and try to copy the quantities they eat.

Q. Do I have to buy all the different types of nuts and lentils?
No, they are just for variety. You can stay with one variety of nuts (Brazil nuts are best) or lentils or replace lentils with aduki beans or mung beans.

Chapter 6
Linda's Internal Cleansing Routine (ICR)

This is the routine which I developed after experimenting on myself. I followed it for three months, and my tummy was significantly flatter afterwards (I could see my toes). It also helped to make my bowels function better. Despite eating a healthy diet I used to get very constipated sometimes, but I no longer have this problem. As an added bonus, the ICR also got rid of some arthritic swelling and tenderness that had been developing in my finger joints for two years.

Laxatives

The main principle of the ICR is to keep the intestinal contents as soft as possible in order to loosen any embedded matter—and at the same time to bulk them up so that they can sweep this matter away. This involves using a laxative every evening, in combination with a fibre supplement.

Herbal laxatives (known as 'stimulating' laxatives) are not suitable. They work purely by stimulating the colon to work harder, and can cause painful spasms.

The other type of laxative, known as 'osmotic' laxatives, works by increasing the amount of water that stays in your intestinal contents as they pass through you. This produces the required softness.

The most common osmotic laxatives are
- Epsom salts (magnesium sulphate)
- Glauber's salts (sodium sulphate).

Sulphate tends to encourage sulphate-reducing bacteria in the intestines, and for health reasons we are also advised to reduce

Chapter 6

> ### Recipe
>
> The Internal Cleansing Routine is carried out daily at bed-time for three months maximum. You will need
> - a large cup or mug with a capacity of at least 300 ml / 10 fl oz / 1.3 US cup
> - 1 small balloon whisk
> - 1 tea bag: licorice tea (women) or chamomile tea (men)
> - boiling water
> - 1 slightly rounded tablespoon magnesium ascorbate powder or Epsom salts
> - 1 slightly rounded tablespoon whole, unpowdered psyllium husks
>
> Put the tea bag in the cup and half fill with boiling water. Leave for a few minutes to infuse, then remove the tea bag and top up the cup with cold water.
>
> Add the magnesium ascorbate or Epsom salts to the tea and stir to dissolve. Add the psyllium husks, and quickly whisk in to incorporate thoroughly. Drink immediately.

our consumption of sodium-rich items. So although these laxatives are fine for occasional use, I would not personally use them on a daily basis. The substance I chose as my laxative was magnesium ascorbate—a form of vitamin C combined with magnesium. It is not normally used as a laxative, but does have a laxative effect very similar to Epsom salts.

One note of caution. Vitamin C taken at levels of more than one gram per day can raise oestrogen levels in women. If you have been diagnosed with a high-oestrogen condition (these can include ovarian cysts, endometriosis and fibroids, for example) or if you are taking the contraceptive pill or oestrogen replacement therapy, you should use Epsom salts instead of magnesium ascorbate. See Appendix IV for where to get magnesium ascorbate powder.

Psyllium husks

Used in India for thousands of years to prevent constipation (and also added to proprietary constipation remedies in the West) psyllium husks are cheap and absorb up to 100 times their weight in water. This makes them ideal to combine with an osmotic laxative, to produce a soft, bulky stool. For recommended brands, see Appendix IV.

Dysbiosis

If you are concerned about the possibility of dysbiosis (see page 46), you may want to add some herbs to your daily routine. The following herbs help to main a healthy balance of intestinal bacteria if you take them at the end of the day and consume probiotic soy yoghurt in the morning.

- Raw garlic
- Oregano extract
- Clove extract
- Wormwood extract

If raw garlic is prepared as follows, the odour will be minimal.

To prepare raw garlic

Have a glass of water and a teaspoon ready. Carefully peel one clove of raw garlic. Using a sharp knife, cut the garlic lengthwise into slices and then into small cubes, taking care not to crush or bruise the garlic. Put the cubes on the teaspoon, place them on the back of your tongue, and immediately swallow with the aid of the glass of water, as if taking a pill.

The other herbs on the list are available micellized in a

capsule, which can be taken at the same time as your laxative. See Resources in Appendix IV.

Frequently asked questions

Q. Will my bowels become lazy if I take laxatives every day?

People do not seem to find this to be the case when they use the ICR. In my own case, I used to have a history of constipation but this was no longer a problem after doing the ICR for three months.

Q. Do I have to use the recommended teas or can I just use plain hot water?

The recommended teas have helpful weight-loss properties and are soothing for the intestines. However you can use plain hot water if you prefer.

Q. Are the quantities of laxative and psyllium husks exact or can I reduce or increase them?

These quantities are for someone of average height and build. You should take enough to produce a very soft but not liquid stool once or twice a day.

Appendix I
Recipes

Useful equipment
Stick blender, grater, pressure cooker, stir-fry pan, juice extractor.

Weights and measures
Most of the recipes here use measurements by volume (measured in a cup or a measuring jug) rather than by weight. 1 US cup = 235 millilitres (ml). This is just under half a UK pint.

Celery and radish Juice
Use enough fresh celery and radish to produce a small wineglassful of juice when processed with a juice extractor. Dilute the juice 50:50 with water before drinking.

The following basic recipes will be needed as advance preparations for some of the meals in the Seven-Day Meal Plan.

French dressing
    6 tbsp extra virgin olive oil
    2 tbsp lemon juice
    salt substitute and freshly ground black pepper

Beat the ingredients together to make a basic French dressing. You can also add other ingredients such as herbs or some finely chopped spring onion (scallion). Whisk the dressing again just before serving.

Appendix I

Cooking brown rice

Brown rice is much more nutritious than white. It is available from supermarkets and health food stores. You can cook brown rice using the directions on the packet, but this method is my favourite. Use half a cup / 115 ml rice per serving. Pre-soak the rice overnight in at least twice its volume of cold water. Before cooking, drain the rice, add enough boiling water to cover it, bring to the boil then cover the pan tightly with a lid and simmer on the lowest possible heat until tender (about 25 minutes). By now the water should all have been absorbed. If not, drain the rice in a sieve and replace it immediately in the pan. Replace the lid and leave the rice in the covered pan away from the heat for five minutes, after which it is ready to serve.

Once cold, brown rice can be spread out on an oiled baking tray, frozen, then crumbled into grains and bagged for the freezer.

Dried beans and chick peas

These are rich in protein and B vitamins. Beans should be soaked in water before use. Cover with four times their volume in boiling water and leave overnight.

Pressure cooking method (fast)

This method is best for chick peas and larger beans. Aduki and mung beans can be cooked in a saucepan.

Throw away the soaking water, place the beans, well covered with fresh boiling water, in a pressure cooker, bring to full steam, and leave on a low-to-medium heat for 4-10 minutes, depending on size and age. Remove the pressure cooker from the heat and place it in a sink of cold water. You cannot open the pressure cooker until it has cooled down enough to reduce the steam pressure inside. Remove the lid and cut a bean to ensure that it is tender. If not, return the beans to the pan and cook for a little longer.

Saucepan method (slower)

Throw away the soaking water, place the beans, well covered with fresh boiling water, in a saucepan, bring back to the boil and boil the beans fast for at least 10 minutes. Then turn down the heat and simmer until tender. This takes approx 30-50 minutes for aduki beans and mung beans, and an hour or more for larger beans and chick peas.

To freeze, allow to cool and follow the same method as for frozen brown rice.

Lentils

A quantity of lentils can be prepared in advance and will keep in the fridge for up to 4 days, or can be frozen. They are rich in protein, B vitamins and iron.

Use half a cup / 115 ml uncooked lentils per serving. Put the lentils in a large pan and add about 2½ times their volume of boiling water plus a tablespoon of olive oil to stop them frothing up too much. Never add salt at this stage, as it will toughen them. Bring to the boil and simmer for 25-40 minutes, depending on the size and age of the lentils. Stir occasionally. Red lentils take only 25 minutes. Brown, green or yellow lentils take 30 to 40 minutes. Lentils boil over easily, which is why it is a good idea to use a pan several sizes larger than you would normally need.

To freeze cooked lentils, allow them to cool and put spoonfuls in the wells of tart or muffin baking tins. Freeze the tins then empty out the frozen lentils, put them in bags and return to the freezer.

Recipes for the Seven-Day Meal Plan

Please see the chart on pages 66-67 for the full meal plan. These recipes only cover the items that require preparation or cooking.

Monday Lunch

Salad of roasted peppers, tomatoes and courgettes (zucchini)

For each serving
    1 red or green (bell) pepper, deseeded and quartered
    2 tomatoes, halved
    1 medium courgette (zucchini), cut lengthwise in half and then into 2-inch segments
    4 tbsp olive oil
    1 tbsp balsamic vinegar
    A thumb-sized piece of orange or lemon peel, finely shredded with a sharp knife

Preheat oven to 400F/200C/Gas 6. Put the vegetable pieces and shredded peel on an oiled baking tray, brush with 2 tbsp olive oil, and place the baking tray in the oven for 30 minutes or until the vegetables are tender and beginning to brown.

When cooked, remove from the oven, allow to cool, then toss in a bowl with the balsamic vinegar and the remaining olive oil. Season with salt substitute and freshly ground black pepper.

Monday Dinner

Yellow lentil, potato and cauliflower soup with coriander, spiced with curry powder

For each serving
    1 cup / 235 ml cooked yellow lentils (see page 78)
    2 handfuls cauliflower florets, cut small
    1 medium potato, diced
    1 tbsp coriander (cilantro), chopped
    1 tbsp lemon juice
    2 tsp curry powder (ensure it contains turmeric)
    boiling water

Put the potato and cauliflower in a saucepan and add enough boiling water to barely cover the vegetables. Bring the pan to the boil, cover and simmer gently for 15 minutes or until tender.

Stir the curry powder into the cooked lentils and then add the mixture to the saucepan. Stir, return the pan to boiling point and immediately remove from the heat. Season with salt substitute then finally stir in the chopped coriander (cilantro) and serve.

Tuesday Lunch

Chickpea salad with parsley, chopped celery, chopped red onion and French dressing

For each serving
    1 cup / 235 ml recently-cooked (still warm) chick peas (see page 77)
    1 stick celery, thinly sliced
    half a small red onion, thinly sliced
    3 tbsp French dressing (see page 76)
    1 tbsp parsley, chopped

Combine all the ingredients, and season with salt substitute and freshly ground black pepper.

Tuesday Dinner

Broad bean, broccoli and chicken soup

For each serving
    1 cup / 235 ml fresh or frozen broad beans
    2 handfuls broccoli florets, cut small
    1 handful cooked chicken, shredded
    boiling water

If using fresh broad beans, they may have a tough outer skin unless they are young. If so, prepare them as follows. Put the beans in a saucepan of boiling water, bring back to the boil, and drain at once into a colander. Refresh under cold water and leave to cool and dry a little. Pinch each bean to remove the skin and reveal the bright green centre. Discard the skins.

Put the frozen or prepared beans in a saucepan, and pour in just enough boiling water to cover them. Put a lid on the pan, bring back to the boil and simmer gently for a few minutes until tender. Remove the pan from the heat. Using a stick blender, whizz the beans in their water until you have a smooth purée. Add the broccoli florets, return to a medium heat, and cook for a further five minutes or until the broccoli is just tender. Stir in the shredded chicken, gently heat through, season with salt substitute and freshly ground black pepper, and serve.

Appendix I

Wednesday Lunch

Salad of cooked brown rice tossed with French dressing, chopped parsley, celery, red and green peppers

For each serving
- 1 cup /235 ml cooked brown rice (see page 77)
- 1 stick celery, thinly sliced
- half a red sweet (bell) pepper, thinly sliced
- half a green sweet (bell) pepper, thinly sliced
- 3 tbsp French dressing
- 1 tsp parsley, chopped

Combine all the ingredients and season with salt substitute and freshly-ground black pepper.

Wednesday Dinner

Green lentil soup with white fish, cabbage, ginger and chives

For each serving
    1 cup / 235 ml cooked green lentils
    4 oz / 115 grams white fish, filleted and cut into bite-sized chunks
    1 handful green cabbage, finely shredded
    1 thumb-sized piece of fresh ginger, finely chopped
    1 tbsp lemon juice
    1 tsp chives, chopped
    Boiling water

Put the cooked lentils in a saucepan and stir in enough boiling water to produce a soupy but not watery consistency. Stir in the shredded cabbage and ginger and bring to the boil over a medium heat. Simmer gently for five minutes, stirring occasionally, then season with salt substitute and add the chives and fish pieces. Return the pan to the heat, bring back to boiling point and immediately remove from the heat. Cover the pan and leave for two minutes. Check that the fish is cooked through (it should flake easily) and serve.

Thursday lunch

Aduki bean salad with parsley, chopped celery, tomato and French dressing

For each serving
    1 cup / 235 ml aduki beans (or from a can, rinsed in boiling water and thoroughly drained)
    2 medium tomatoes, skinned, deseeded and roughly chopped
    1 stick celery, thinly sliced
    3 tbsp French dressing
    1 tsp parsley, chopped

Tomato skins should slip off easily if you put the tomatoes in a bowl of boiling water and remove after 30 seconds. Cut the tomatoes in half crosswise and scoop out the seeds before chopping.

Gently combine the ingredients and season with salt substitute and freshly-ground black pepper.

Thursday Dinner

Red lentil soup with broccoli and chicken

For each serving
    1 cup / 235 ml cooked red lentils
    2 handfuls broccoli florets, cut small
    1 handful cooked chicken, shredded
    1 tbsp lemon juice
    boiling water

Put the cooked lentils in a saucepan and stir in just enough boiling water to produce a soupy but not watery consistency. Stir in the broccoli florets and bring to the boil over a medium heat. Simmer gently for 5 minutes, stirring occasionally. Stir in the shredded chicken. Bring back to the boil, season with salt substitute and freshly-ground black pepper, then remove from the heat and serve.

Friday lunch

Prawns (shrimps) in egg-free mayonnaise with salad of cooked brown rice tossed with chopped parsley, celery, grated radish and French dressing

For each serving
- half a cup / 115 ml cooked, peeled prawns (shrimps)
- 1 generous tbsp egg-free mayonnaise (from health-food store)
- 1 cup / 235 ml cooked brown rice
- 2 radishes, grated
- 1 stick celery, thinly sliced
- 3 tbsp French dressing
- 1 tsp parsley, chopped

Combine the prawns with the mayonnaise, season with freshly-ground black pepper and put to one side. Combine the remaining ingredients, and season with salt substitute and freshly-ground black pepper.

Friday Dinner

Mung bean soup with onion, garlic and tofu chunks

For each serving
    1 cup / 235 ml cooked mung beans
    4 oz / 125 g firm tofu (not the 'silken' variety)
    1 medium onion, cut in half lengthwise then thinly sliced
    1 clove garlic
    3 tbsp olive oil
    1 tbsp lemon juice
    boiling water

Cut the tofu into bite-sized chunks and fry in the olive oil over a medium heat on both sides until golden. Put to one side. Crush the garlic clove with the flat side of a knife then peel and chop it. In the same oil, sweat the sliced onion over a medium heat until tender, then add the chopped garlic and put to one side. Reserve 1 large tbsp of the mung beans and put to one side. Pour just enough boiling water on the remaining beans to allow you to process them to a medium-thick soup consistency with a stick blender. Now stir in the remaining beans plus the tofu, onion and garlic and bring back to the boil gently over a medium heat, stirring occasionally. Season with salt substitute and freshly-ground black pepper and serve.

Appendix I

Saturday Brunch

Smoothie

For each serving
1 cup / 235 ml soy milk
half an avocado pear
1 level tbsp ground almonds (almond flour)
1 handful fresh or frozen berries
Whizz in a blender until smooth. Drink immediately otherwise the avocado may spoil.

Kedgeree

For each serving
    1 cup / 235 ml cold cooked brown rice
    4 oz / 125 g fresh haddock fillet
    half a cup / 115 ml fresh or frozen peas
    2 tbsp olive oil
    1 tbsp parsley, chopped
    boiling water

Put the peas in a saucepan, just covered with boiling water and bring back to the boil over a medium heat. Simmer until tender, then drain into a sieve or colander. Put the haddock fillet in a stir-fry pan with a few tablespoons of water, cover the pan, bring it to the boil, turn down the heat to the lowest setting and simmer very gently for a few minutes until the fish flakes easily. Remove the fish from the pan and put to one side. Now add the olive oil to the same pan, followed by the rice. Turn the heat up to medium and stir-fry the rice to heat it through. Flake the fish, then gently fold in the fish, peas and parsley. Season with salt substitute and freshly ground pepper then serve.

Saturday Dinner

Thai chicken curry

For each serving
- 1 raw chicken breast, cut into thin strips
- 1/2 cup / 115 ml mixed chopped frozen vegetables (e.g. corn kernels, peppers, carrots)
- generous 3/4 cup or 200 ml canned coconut milk
- 60 g / 2 oz fine dried rice noodles or vermicelli
- 2 tbsp groundnut oil
- 1 tsp red Thai curry paste

Heat the groundnut oil in a stir-fry pan over a medium heat, add the chicken strips and stir-fry until golden. Remove from the pan and put to one side. Add the curry paste to the same pan, stir briefly then pour in the coconut milk, followed by the chopped vegetables and the cooked chicken. Bring to the boil and simmer gently, stirring, until the vegetables are tender and the chicken cooked through. Meanwhile put the rice noodles in a bowl and cover with boiling water to soften for a few minutes. Drain thoroughly in a sieve, place in a serving dish and stir in the rice milk, chicken and vegetables. Season with salt substitute and serve.

Rice pudding

(2-3 servings)
    1/2 cup / 115 ml short-grain brown rice
    4 cups / 1 litre soy milk
    1 tsp good quality vanilla extract
    1 pinch cinnamon
    4 tbsp brown rice (malt) syrup
    4 tbsp raisins
Preheat the oven to 275C/140F/gas 1.

Mix all the ingredients in a saucepan, bring to the boil over a medium heat and simmer gently for 20 minutes, stirring occasionally. Transfer to an ovenproof dish, cover and bake for 1 hour or until the pudding has set.

If using cooked fruit, select your fresh or frozen fruit, chop into bite-sized pieces if necessary, place in a separate oven-proof dish, cover it tightly and cook in the oven along with the rice. Serve the fruit spooned over the rice.

Sunday Brunch

Smoothie: see recipe for Saturday brunch

Fish fillet fried in olive oil with grilled/broiled courgettes (zucchini) and tomatoes

For each serving
    1 x 4 oz / 120 g fish fillet per person
    2 medium courgettes (zucchini) cut in half lengthwise
    two medium tomatoes, cut in half
    3 tbsp olive oil

Preheat the grill (broiler). Brush the courgettes and tomatoes with olive oil and place under the grill. Cook until beginning to brown. Remove the tomatoes. Turn the courgettes over to brown the other side. Heat the rest of the olive oil in a frying pan (skillet) over a medium heat. When the oil is sizzling, add the fish and cook on both sides until done. The time varies according to the thickness of the fish, but it is cooked when it flakes easily. Do not overcook. Season the fish and vegetables

Appendix I

Sunday Dinner

Gluten-free pasta bake with salmon and roasted vegetables

For two servings
    4 oz / 120 g gluten-free pasta (corn, rice, millet etc.)
    4 oz / 120 g fresh salmon fillet
    1 medium red onion, cut into quarters
    1 medium courgette (zucchini) cut in half lengthwise, then into chunks
    1 medium green (bell) pepper, cut into thick slices
    Olive oil

Preheat oven to 200C/400F/Gas 6. Put the vegetable pieces on an oiled baking tray, brush them with olive oil, and place the baking tray in the oven for 30 minutes or until the vegetables are tender and beginning to brown. Remove from the oven and put to one side. Turn the oven down to 350F/180C/gas 4.

Cook the pasta as directed on the packet. When cooked, drain it and toss in 2 tbsp olive oil. Poach the salmon for a few minutes in a lidded saucepan in a few tablespoons of water over a low heat. The salmon is done when it flakes easily. Drain the salmon, flake it and combine in a bowl with the pasta and vegetables. Season with salt substitute and freshly-ground black pepper. Transfer to an oven-proof dish, cover tightly with tin foil and place in the oven for 30 minutes before serving.

This dish can also be prepared in advance and placed in the oven at the last minute.

Tofu chocolate mousse

For each serving
    4 oz / 120 g silken tofu
    1 level tbsp cocoa powder
    1 tbsp brown rice (malt) syrup
    A few drops of good quality vanilla extract

Small quantities are best prepared with a stick blender. Put all the ingredients in a suitable container and blend until smooth and creamy. (This may take a few minutes of blending.)

Appendix II
Vitamins A and D

People who know me know that I frequently issue warnings about two nutritional deficiencies which I believe are becoming very common due to dieting and health-conscious eating habits.

Nowadays, most diet-conscious adults consume low-fat versions of foods like milk, cheese and yoghurt. If they are dairy-intolerant, they may even avoid these foods completely. It's good for adults to control the amount of fats they consume. But on the other hand, if you avoid dairy fats, you are also avoiding virtually the only dietary sources of vitamins A and D (apart from liver and some types of fish).

Vitamin A

If you think you can get plenty of vitamin A from the beta carotene found in carrots and other vegetables, think again. You have to eat an awful lot of beta carotene just to make a little vitamin A. And beta carotene can only be absorbed and converted when enough fat or oil is present in the same meal.

Strenuous physical exercise, too much alcohol, too much iron (especially from processed foods which have been 'fortified' with iron) excessive polyunsaturated fats, or zinc deficiency can also reduce the amount of vitamin A which your body is able to make from beta carotene.

Children can only make a little vitamin A from beta carotene. Babies, and people with diabetes or poor thyroid function cannot make vitamin A at all.

So it can be unwise to depend on plant sources for vitamin A. This vital nutrient is needed for the growth and repair of body tissues. It protects against acne, aids digestion and helps to build strong bones and teeth. It is essential for good eyesight and helps to prevent infections—for instance children with vitamin A deficiency are more prone to getting measles. Vitamin A deficiency in pregnant mothers results in offspring with eye defects, harelip, cleft palate and abnormalities of the heart and blood vessels.

Vitamin D

Sometimes known as the 'sunshine vitamin' vitamin D may also be very low in the diets of people who avoid dairy products or eat low-fat versions of these foods. Your body can make some vitamin D from sunshine, but in northern countries such as the UK, the right light particles for this are only present for a few months of the year.

People with the highest risk of vitamin D deficiency are those who use sunscreen products on their skin or rarely go outdoors. Many elderly people are at risk, and also people in institutions such as prisons. Research from the Harvard School of Public Health shows that supplementing elderly people with vitamin D considerably reduces their risk of falling.

Science is now revealing that auto-immune diseases such as multiple sclerosis are virtually confined to relatively northern countries. Scientists believe that this is due to a lack of vitamin D.

An autoimmune disease is one where the body's tissues become damaged due to chronic inflammation. Cells involved in inflammation should die once their job is done. When insufficient vitamin D is present, it seems that these cells do not get the signal to die. So the inflammation can continue until it is eventually diagnosed as an auto-immune disease such as multiple sclerosis, rheumatoid arthritis or thyroiditis. (The name given depends on where the damage occurs— nerves, joints, thyroid gland and so on).

If you are overweight due to low thyroid function, you should get checked for autoimmune thyroiditis. Very often this condition goes undiagnosed and doctors simply hand out thyroid replacement hormones.

If you have trouble exercising because your muscles feel weak and don't seem to strengthen easily, this may also be due to vitamin D deficiency.

Soy foods help the body convert vitamin D to its active form.

Cod liver oil

The one supplement which I recommend more than any other (except perhaps vitamin C) is cod liver oil. Rich in both vitamin A and D, this is the perfect supplement for people who are at risk of deficiency.

Appendix III
Testing for problem foods

If you lost a lot of weight very quickly during the initial four weeks of the Flat Stomach Diet, it is likely that you have water retention and need to test yourself to find out if you have any problem foods (see page 59). Otherwise your water weight will come back when you deviate from the diet, and you will not know why. The same applies to any bloating relief which the diet achieved for you.

The test takes four weeks. During this time you must continue to avoid all foods in List B on page 64—with one exception. Under controlled conditions you will also—one at a time—eat the foods which are starred as 'potential triggers of bloating or water retention'. These foods are candidates for causing these problems and have to be tested at the rate of one per week as described below. This test only works when you have not consumed these foods for several weeks.

Procedure

Week 1 WHEAT TEST	Continue avoiding all 'NO' foods, except for egg-free wheat pasta, wheat flour or plain wheat crackers. Eat one of these foods every day for 5 days, then stop. If you get any unpleasant reactions, such as headaches, sinus congestion or drowsiness, or if your weight rises by several pounds during that time, make a note of them and stop eating the wheat before the 5 days is up. There is no point in continuing, because it is likely that wheat is a problem food for you and you need to continue avoiding it. Whether or not you experience a reaction, stop the wheat after 5 days, and avoid all the 'NO' foods for the next 2 days.
Week 2 DAIRY TEST	Repeat what you did in Wk 1, consuming cow's milk products daily instead of wheat: fresh milk, cheese and yoghurt. The procedure is exactly the same as for Wk 1.
Week 3 EGGS TEST	Repeat what you did in Wk 1, consuming eggs daily instead of wheat. If you do not want to eat a whole egg every day, make a 2-egg omelette with plain egg and water, cook it very thinly, and eat a small strip each day for the test period.
Week 4 YEAST TEST	Repeat what you did in Wk 1, consuming yeast daily instead of wheat. Buy a small jar of low-sodium yeast extract from a health food store, and make it into a hot drink with boiling water. Drink this each day for the test period.

After the test you can safely resume eating those foods which did not provoke any symptoms such as fatigue, headaches or water retention. But do continue to avoid any foods which tested positive.

Read all labels carefully. A few crumbs a day can undo your hard work

Appendix IV: Resources

Youtube videos of some short, simple Pilates routines

Quick Abdominal Exercise Routine: Lorie Baker's Pilates Routine
http://bit.ly/8pH0t
More Advanced: Diethealth's Pilates Core Workout Video
http://bit.ly/2lUYqg

Or get this recommended DVD for a full Pilates workout

From Amazon.co.uk: http://amzn.ws/pilatesdvd-uk
From Amazon.com: http://lose-pounds.net/category/pilates-dvds/

Foods, Herbs and Supplements

UNITED KINGDOM

Recommended sweetener

Some UK supermarkets and health food stores sell organic Clearspring brown rice (malt) syrup. Try looking in the 'Free From' section. Otherwise you can order it online here:
http://amzn.ws/clearspring-maltsyrup-uk

Supplements and herbal products

Micellised oregano, clove, wormwood extract
http://amzn.ws/oreganocomplex-uk
Bromelain: http://amzn.ws/bromelain-uk
Magnesium ascorbate powder
http://amzn.ws/magascorbate-powder-uk
Agnus castus: http://amzn.ws/agnuscastus-uk
Deglycerrized licorice capsules

Appendix IV

http://amzn.ws/licorice-deglyccaps-uk
Licorice teabags: http://amzn.ws/licoriceteabags-uk
Spice teabags (cinnamon, cloves, cardamom, ginger) http://amzn.ws/cinnamonspicetea-uk
Psyllium husks: http://amzn.ws/psylliumhusks-uk
Juice extractor: http://amzn.ws/juiceextractor-uk

Suppliers of gluten-free foods

Many of these brands are available in supermarkets such as Sainsburys
Clearspring, www.clearspring.co.uk
Doves Organic, www.dovesfarm.co.uk
Eat Natural, www.eatnatural.co.uk
Health Link UK www.healthlinkuk.com
Natures Path, www.naturespath.com
Orgran, www.orgran.com
Real Foods, www.realfoods.co.uk
Virginia Harvest, www.virginiafoods.net

UNITED STATES

Recommended sweeteners

Some UK supermarkets and health food stores sell organic Clearspring brown rice (malt) syrup. Try looking in the 'Free From' section. Otherwise you can order it online here:
http://amzn.ws/clearspring-maltsyrup-uk

Supplements and herbal products

Black walnut, cloves, wormwood
http://amzn.ws/wormwoodclovesformula-us
Bromelain: http://amzn.ws/jarrow-bromelain-us
Magnesium ascorbate powder
http://amzn.ws/magascorbate-powder-us

Agnus castus: http://amzn.ws/agnuscastus-us
Deglycerrized licorice capsules
http://amzn.ws/licorice-deglyccaps-us
Licorice teabags: http://amzn.ws/licoriceteabags-us
Cinnamon teabags: http://amzn.ws/cinnamonspicetea-us
Psyllium husks: http://amzn.ws/psylliumhusks-us
Juice extractor: http://amzn.ws/juiceextractor-us

Suppliers of gluten-free foods

Natures Path, www.naturespath.com
Bob's Red Mill, www.bobsredmill.com
Bakery on Main, www.bakeryonmain.com
U.S. Mills (Erewhon), www.usmillsllc.com
The Better Health Store, www.thebetterhealthstore.com
Gluten Free Mall, www.glutenfreemall.com

More resources

Digital downloads, including factsheets, student materials and Linda's book *Treat Yourself with Nutritional Therapy* with self-help programmes for everything from migraine to arthritis. Includes many recipes suitable for use with Linda's Flat Stomach programme.
www.health-diets.net/downloads/index.html
Printed version of *Treat Yourself with Nutritional Therapy*
www.health-diets.net/books/

The Waterfall Diet

Linda's book on water retention, published by Piatkus books
From Amazon UK: http://amzn.ws/waterfalldietbook-uk
From Amazon.com: http://amzn.ws/waterfalldietbook-us

Visit **www.health-diets.net/flat-stomach/members/** for clickable versions of all the internet links in this book.

A final note

I wish you all success with your flat stomach program and would love to know how you get on. If you haven't already subscribed, you may be interested in signing up for my twice-monthly newsletters. Use this link to subscribe: www.health-diets.net/newsletters.html

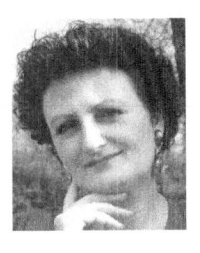

Below is a link to find clickable links to all the resources mentioned in this book, which is useful if you have bought the printed version.
www.health-diets.net/flat-stomach/members/

If you're interested in training to be a naturopathic nutritionist why not check out my other website www.naturostudy.org.

Linda Lazarides

Got an annoying health problem?
Linda can write you a personal Health & Diet program to help fix it.
www.health-diets.net/consultations/

Follow Linda Lazarides on Twitter
http://twitter.com/LindaLazarides

Subscribe to Linda's email newsletters
www.health-diets.net/newsletters.html

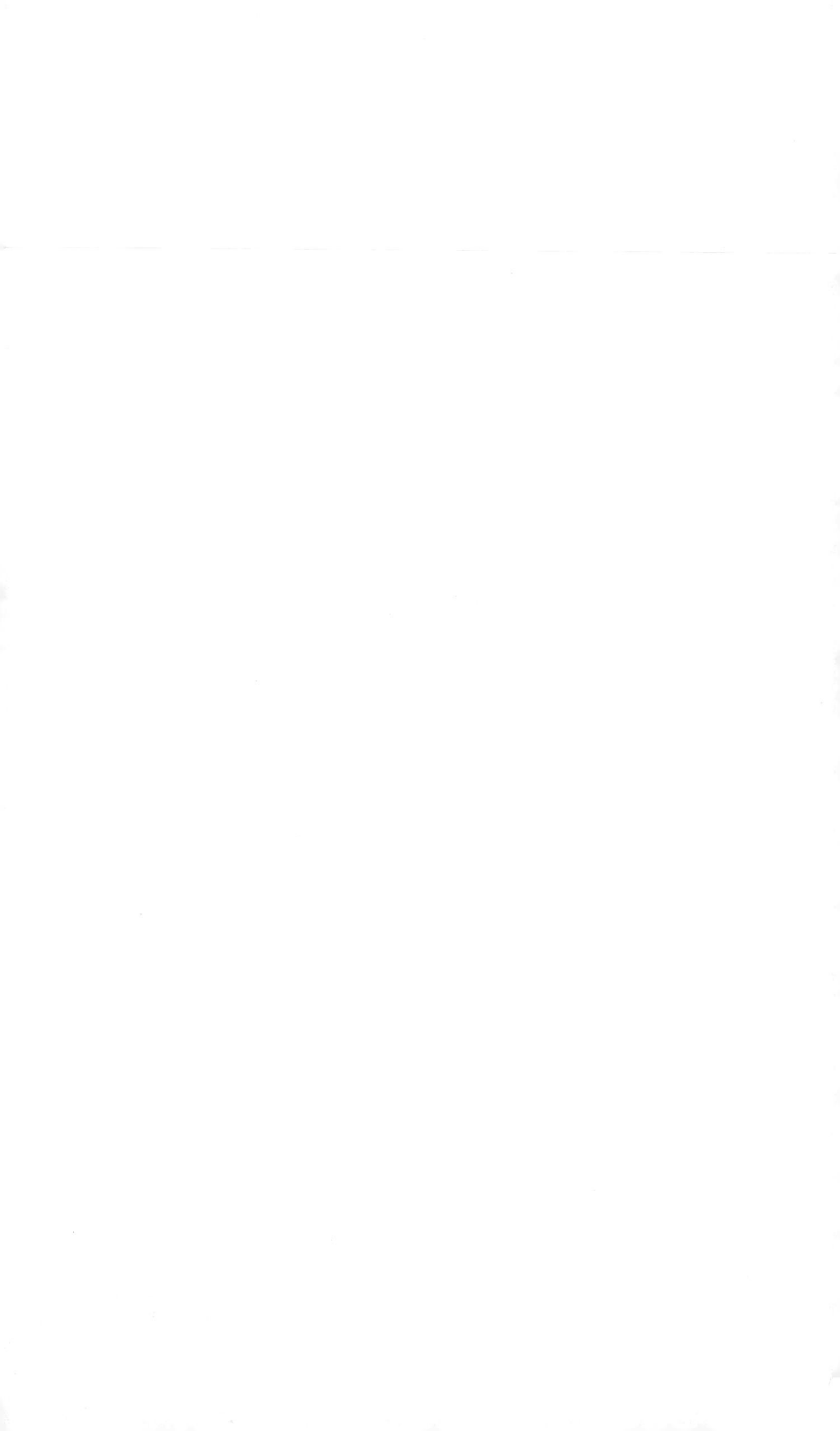